THE Kosmic Kitchen COOKBOOK

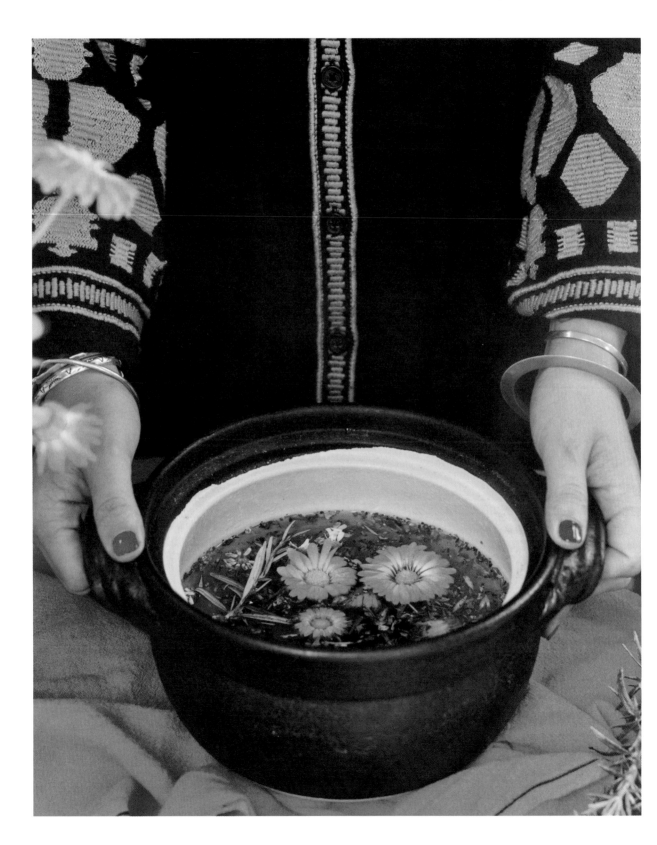

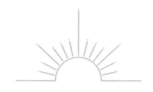

THE

Everyday Herbalism and Recipes

KOSMIC

for Radical Wellness

KITCHEN

Sarah Kate Benjamin & Summer Singletary

WITH PHOTOGRAPHS BY ANNA-ALEXIA BASILE

COOKBOOK

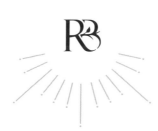

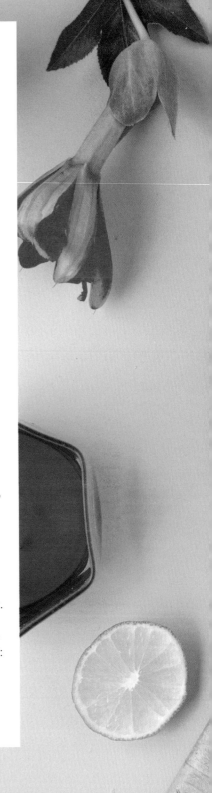

Roost Books
An imprint of Shambhala Publications, Inc.
2129 13th Street
Boulder, Colorado 80302
roostbooks.com

Cover photography: Anna-Alexia Basile
Cover and title page lettering: Alicia Schultz
Cover and interior design: Amy Sly
Stylist: Alysia Andriola

9 8 7 6 5 4 3

Printed in China

♾ This edition is printed on acid-free paper that meets the
American National Standards Institute Z39.48 Standard.
♻ Shambhala Publications makes every effort to print on
postconsumer recycled paper. For more information please
visit www.shambhala.com.
Roost Books is distributed worldwide by Penguin Random House, Inc.,
and its subsidiaries.

Library of Congress Cataloging-in-Publication Data
Names: Benjamin, Sarah Kate, author. | Singletary, Summer
Ashley, author.
Title: The Kosmic kitchen cookbook: everyday herbalism and recipes
for radical wellness / Sarah Kate Benjamin, Summer Ashley Singletary.
Description: Boulder: Roost Books, 2020. | Includes index.
Identifiers: LCCN 2019028298 | ISBN 9781611807141 (trade paperback)
Subjects: LCSH: Natural foods. | Cooking. | Food. | Nutrition. | LCGFT:
Cookbooks.
Classification: LCC TX369 .B47 2020 | DDC 641.3/02—dc23
LC record available at https://lccn.loc.gov/2019028298

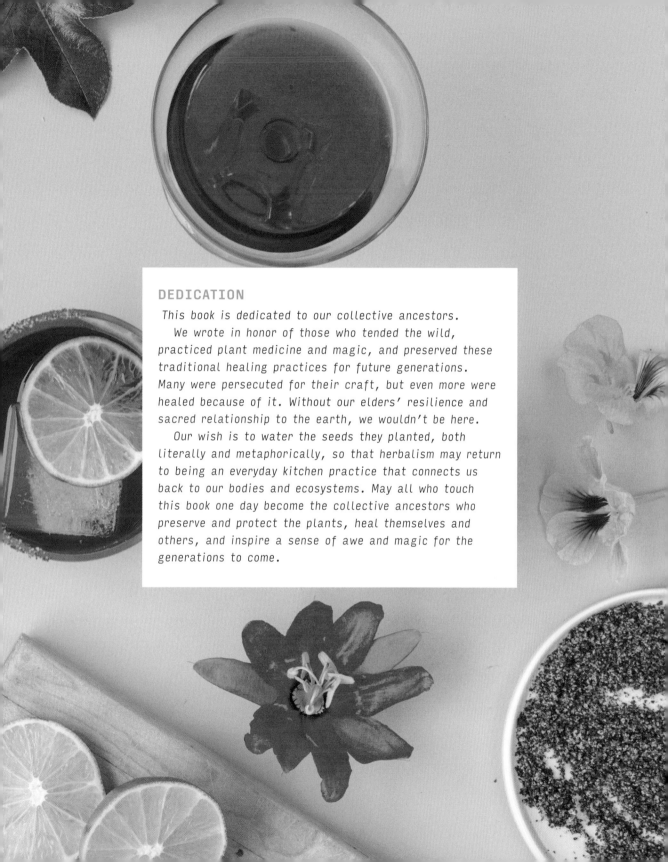

DEDICATION

This book is dedicated to our collective ancestors.

We wrote in honor of those who tended the wild, practiced plant medicine and magic, and preserved these traditional healing practices for future generations. Many were persecuted for their craft, but even more were healed because of it. Without our elders' resilience and sacred relationship to the earth, we wouldn't be here.

Our wish is to water the seeds they planted, both literally and metaphorically, so that herbalism may return to being an everyday kitchen practice that connects us back to our bodies and ecosystems. May all who touch this book one day become the collective ancestors who preserve and protect the plants, heal themselves and others, and inspire a sense of awe and magic for the generations to come.

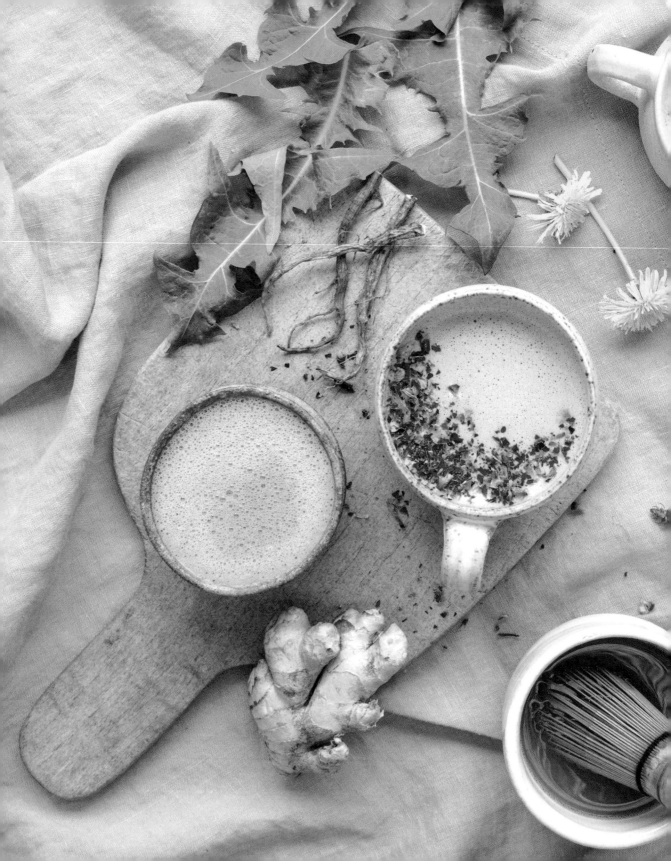

CONTENTS

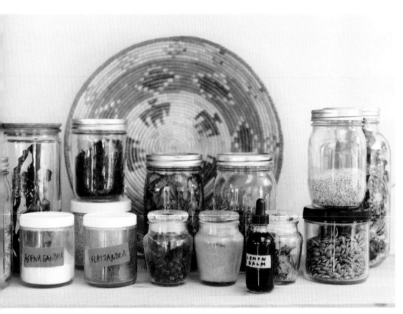

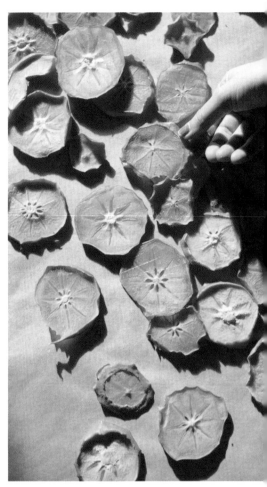

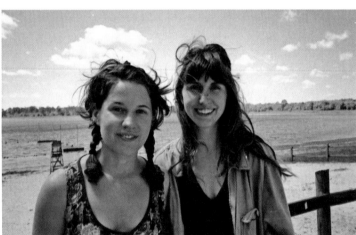

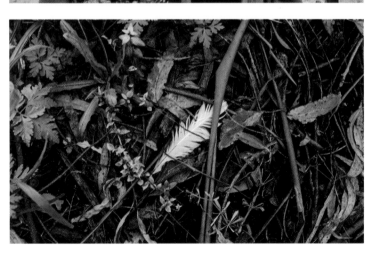

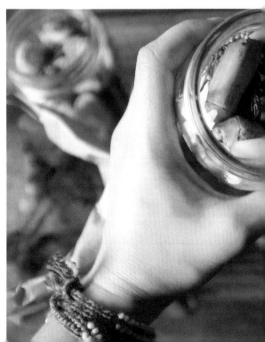

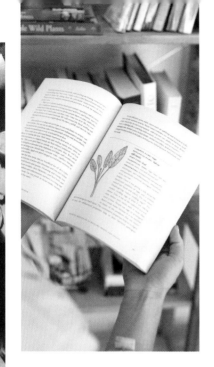

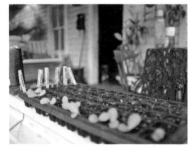

Introduction

The Kosmic Kitchen began from a friendship planted in a community garden in the lush, green backdrop of central Florida. Growing food and herbs together in our campus garden is where we first connected with nourishment practices. It wasn't long before we started experimenting with the garden's bounty of wild weeds and aromatic herbs in our kitchen. Because of the semitropical ecosystem, we were able to grow almost anything. We regularly incorporated fresh tulsi, catnip, chamomile, calendula, Cuban oregano, hibiscus, lemon balm, and passionflower. With these new smells wafting from the stove, our friends took notice too. We didn't host your average dinner party; we enjoyed meals on the front porch of our bungalow, cooked food we had growing in the front yard garden, and infused everything we could with medicinal herbs.

Both of us grew up in Florida, but it wasn't until we started to grow our own food and learn about the plants living alongside us that our world began to open, the plants becoming a way to connect to our home as well as to ourselves and our community. Growing food and herbs to feed our loved ones is one of the richest human experiences, and since we learn by direct experience, we thought, what better way to learn about plant properties or food as medicine than to eat together?

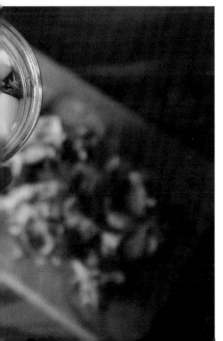

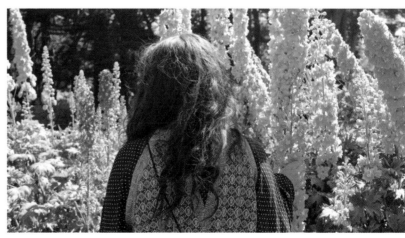

We deepened our work in herbalism by studying with our mentor and friend, Emily Ruff, at the Florida School of Holistic Living in Orlando, Florida. Emily opened the door to herbalism for us and expanded our community of people with a kindred curiosity about the healing plant kingdom. What we love about Emily's approach to teaching is that she makes herbalism accessible in urban environments. We didn't need to escape to the country or join a commune (though that would be fun too) to learn about plants and practice herbalism. Her focus is on using what you have, quite literally, growing around you—from wild weeds such as gotu kola and bidens to native and southern plant varieties such as beautyberry and horsemint.

Collectively, we've studied herbalism in Peru, Vermont, and Oregon, and eventually we landed in California together. We've been lucky enough to study with some amazing people too—Rosemary Gladstar, David Hoffmann, Candis Cantin, DeAnna Batdorff, Mark Disharoon, and Kathleen Harrison, to name a few of our teachers.

The Kosmic Kitchen officially began as a Tumblr in 2012 that served as a journal between friends, a place where we shared herbal recipes from our gardens with our local community. It has since grown into a large online community of plant lovers who believe in the power of plants and their capacity to heal. Our vision has grown too. We work to spread the idea of a kosmic kitchen, so folks begin to see their own kitchen as a healing sanctuary full of plant remedies, much like our ancestors did. We believe a kosmic kitchen is a place to reconnect to ourselves, the plants, and nature's elemental processes. We hope that each person who finds this book feels inspired to connect with the magic that's all around us by using plants to create healing rituals each day.

Our Healing Journeys

A big part of how we arrived here is through crisis. While we were growing food and herbs in our gardens, we were both dealing with major health issues. We believe the plants called us to do this work and healed us through the process. Each time we teach a workshop, we share these stories as a way to connect with those who are struggling. The plants and practices you find healing might be different, but these stories are meant to inspire hope and possibility in times that can often feel bleak.

In the midst of marketing and the influencer age, it's easy to feel pressured to be healthy and vibrant. Sometimes we even felt shame and guilt around our illnesses. At times, chronic fatigue syndrome and irritable bowel syndrome (IBS) prevented us from enjoying many foods, hanging out with friends, and being as seemingly carefree as others. But without the dark days there is no light. These challenging times helped us discover our boundaries, learn more about our needs, and ultimately learn that our bodies have an innate desire to heal and can do so even after incredible trauma.

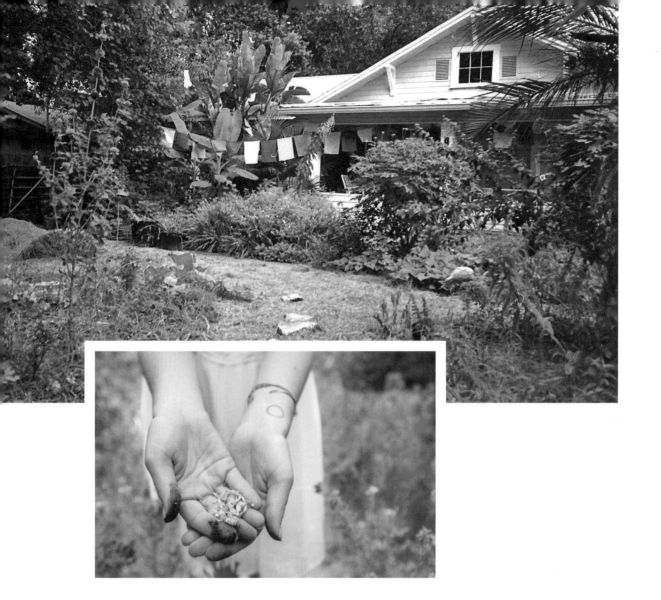

Many of us feel pressure to maintain the illusion that everything is OK. We found that as we began to be more vocal and transparent about our challenges, we found help when we needed it most. We urge you to take the time and space you need to heal and invest in the therapies you feel are necessary for recovery. And if you're feeling well, advocate for and invest in the well-being of your community.

Herbalism and traditional medicine aren't just practices for the well and affluent, though this is what is often represented in media. These plant-based practices are health care, a human right. Outside much of the Western world, herbalism is commonplace and known as the peoples' medicine, passed down through the generations and based on plants specific to the local bioregion. In this time of climate and political crisis, an herbal revolution is breaking through the pavement. Let's heal together and dream a new future where kitchen and community herbalism is commonplace and accessible to all.

Summer's Healing Story

I first fell in love with plants through gardening. The garden was a place I felt hopeful, and the more I learned about plants, the more convinced I became that these beings have healing potential for us all. By watching the cycles of the seasons within the garden, I realized that everything has the power to regenerate in some form or another. The garden felt like a safe haven away from the stress of college and my rather sobering degree in environmental studies, which highlighted the very real consequences of human-led climate change.

Around this time, I was struggling with IBS. This condition basically means that nobody truly knows what's wrong with you, but your brain and gut are having some serious communication issues. It leads to every digestive upset imaginable: bloating, gas, constipation, diarrhea—need I say more? My symptoms were always linked to stress. After I ate anything, I would immediately need to use the restroom and was doubled over in pain. I had to schedule my life around my eating times. I became desperate to heal, and doctors of the time offered no real solutions.

I started to eliminate foods, relationships, and practices that weren't serving me. I even stopped taking birth control, just to see what it would feel like to let my body run its own natural rhythms, and my period stopped coming altogether for the next eight months.

I was incredibly scared and convinced that something was very wrong with me. My doctor told me that there wasn't much that could be done for my IBS systematically, and my gynecologist suggested that I just get back on the pill. I was in the midst of my first healing crisis and my intuition guided me to grow even closer to the plants.

I threw myself into my work in a community garden program. When I told Tina, my mentor and the herbalist who ran the garden at the university, about my health concerns, she suggested I look into vitex berries. They (not so) coincidentally were in season at the time, and I had already been collecting the berries from the tree in our community garden. Amazingly enough, after just a month of taking vitex each day, my period returned. This experience always reminds me of an old herbal adage that says the medicine you need is often right outside your door.

After that, I dedicated myself to the plants. I found medicines such as skullcap and chamomile to calm my frayed nerves, marshmallow root to soothe the inflammation in my gut, raspberry leaf to balance my menstrual cycle, and adaptogens such as tulsi and ashwagandha to restore my endocrine system. Sarah and I started studying ecosystems through permaculture and learned how the relationships between plants and people can work together in a harmonious system.

I also began to intuitively connect with plants by sitting with them and making medicines in accordance with the moon, a practice taught to me by our mentor Emily Ruff. Over time, I realized that much like eating seasonally, herbalism

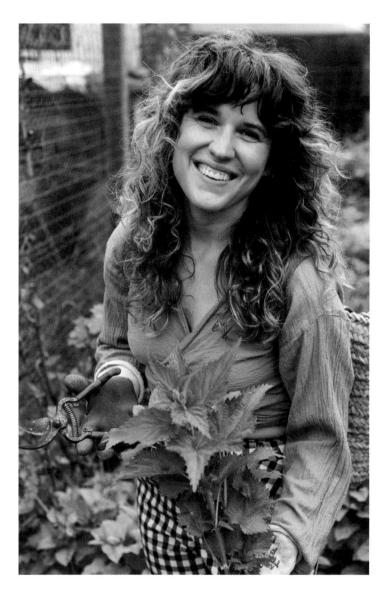

was best practiced in accordance with the seasons and the plants growing around you. Herbalism, as it turns out, is quite intuitive; you just have to be in communication with the living green world around you.

As I continued my studies and my healing journey, I spent a summer at Sage Mountain, an herbal retreat center and botanical sanctuary, interning and studying under Rosemary Gladstar, which was a highlight of my life. She's considered to be the godmother of Western herbalism, as she was a part of the spark the led its revival here in the seventies, and since then has spearheaded multiple initiatives to advocate for herbalists' rights and organizations such as United Plant Savers to protect and preserve North American herbs. At the time I feared that I would not be a good herbalist if I could not heal myself. Rosemary lovingly chuckled and reminded me that so many of us have been called to the healing path due to illness. These extreme experiences help us develop compassion and wisdom for those suffering from a similar fate.

I feel so grateful to have experienced not one but a few healing crises, as they led me to plants and a community of plant-loving people and healers. I hope that this book serves as a reminder that your body has an innate vitality and desire to heal, and the plants are always here to support us.

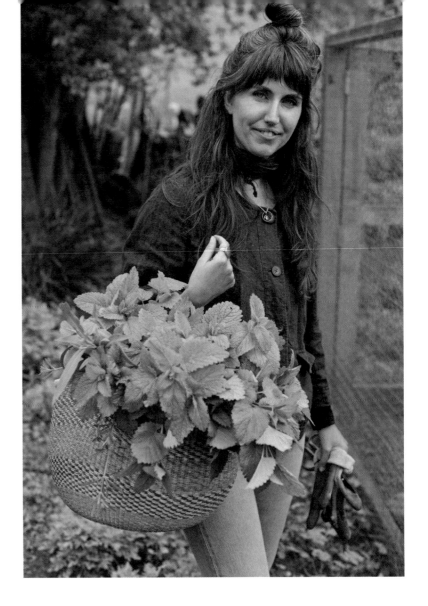

Sarah's Healing Story

My healing story also centers around that community garden. I remember the first time I came across the garden—I immediately felt at home. With Summer, I learned how to grow food and medicinal herbs. At that time, I was craving a sense of community and the garden offered connection in a very deep way. I felt inspired and enlivened by teaching people about the importance of growing food and sustainability practices along with the grounding effect of working with the earth.

If I'm really honest, my first healing crisis started around this time in my life and went on for several years because I didn't give my healing the attention it needed at the time. Being a young woman without the tools to tune in to my body or learn how to truly nourish myself took its toll. I tried veganism and vegetarianism, but I never felt great without animal proteins. I felt depleted and anxious, and I didn't know what my body needed.

After feeling like I had hit rock bottom, I saw a naturopath who diagnosed me with chronic fatigue syndrome. The protocol I was given involved a series of supplements to take at different times of the day, with food and without food—so many pills my head was spinning. Intuitively, I didn't feel that this was the way I was going to heal. Since I was already studying herbalism, I made an appointment with my teacher, Emily Ruff, to get some advice on what to do. She recommended introducing local and organic animal proteins back into my diet, incorporating herbs that supported my adrenals and immune system, and making most of my food at home.

Over the next few months I began looking at my food in a whole new way. When you don't have the energy to cook, or even to get out of bed, it's really hard to nourish yourself. On days when I felt OK, I would prep meals, creating foods such as mineral-rich wild weed pesto, adaptogenic seed-butter bites, immune-boosting bone broths, and herbal-infused salad dressings. I wasn't just cooking anymore. Instead I was making medicine for my meals, and it completely changed the way I ate. Summer and I often hosted dinner parties highlighting these new concoctions, and to our surprise, our friends loved eating this way too and wanted the recipes!

Once I began to feel better, I apprenticed at Herb Pharm, one of the largest US tincture companies. Being surrounded by acres and acres of medicinal plants and working outside gave me more energy than I knew was possible. I was also lucky enough to meet another teacher on this path, Mark Disharoon. He worked side by side in the fields with us, and he taught plant spirit medicine classes each week where we learned about the energetics of plants simply by tasting a few drops of tincture at a time.

It was as if, once again, another door to the plant realm had opened and I was invited to explore the more subtle side of herbal medicine—a place where plants have their own messages, lessons, and ways of healing beyond the physical body. It was then that I began to understand that they too have their own consciousness. Though it isn't easy, I now recognize that every healing crisis serves a certain purpose. There's an inextricable link between the mind, body, and spirit. Physical symptoms are signs of something on a deeper level that is asking to be healed. Plants are really just calling us closer to the ultimate healer, Mother Nature. The more we can learn from the plants, the more we can learn to live in balance with nature and ultimately live in balance with our life.

Where We're Coming From

In this book, we mostly come from the perspectives of Western herbalism (rooted in mostly American and European traditions) and Ayurveda (rooted in the Indian subcontinent and medicine traditions of the region), the modalities we've studied the most over the past decade. As herbalists, we study medicinal plants and how to use them to heal and promote vitality. Ayurveda incorporates herbalism, as do many traditional practices, but it's also an entire system of medicine. Our goal is to awaken you to the power of the elements, but we're not attached to the system(s) you ultimately choose to follow. What's most important is that you tune in to yourself and become aware of life's natural energetic cycles of healing.

Just know that whatever path of practice you choose to follow, it's essential to honor the plants and the places they came from. We believe that to truly heal, we must be activists for more than just ourselves; we must also respect and support the plants as well as the communities who've worked generationally to preserve these ancient traditions. Being an herbalist, *curandera*, shaman, or witch hasn't always been something that could be shared so publicly. Not so long ago, native and marginalized healers and were killed for their beliefs, and healing traditions often went or were forced underground due to colonization.

Modern day herbalism (and our society as a whole) needs serious restructuring from the roots up. In popular culture, certain voices (mainly white) receive more of a platform, while the voices and practices of people of color are underrepresented. Please realize that just because a healing modality, tradition, or healer isn't mainstream, it doesn't discredit the work. Many healers purposefully choose to work locally on a grassroots level, to preserve and protect their craft. And you don't need to go to herb school to be an herbalist! Much of this knowledge is passed down traditionally through stories and experience, and the remedies are made and shared in the kitchen.

We know that we're extremely privileged to be able to share all of these vibrant practices, as this gift is something that was (and still is) fought for. Our hope for this book is to honor these ancient teachings while distilling parts of its vast wisdom to make it more achievable for busy modern lives. Tradition is incredibly important, and we also want to make it clear that this isn't strictly an Ayurvedic or Western herbalism book—we have our own unique twist on things based on our healing journeys and what worked for us. There are many incredible traditional books out there, and we've listed a few in our resources section (page 249) in hopes that you'll be inspired to dive deeper and study with herbal and Ayurvedic practitioners and teachers. Ayurveda is also not our cultural tradition, and we realize there's a responsibility that comes with that, and we understand it to be a living tradition—one that continues as people learn about and use its teachings.

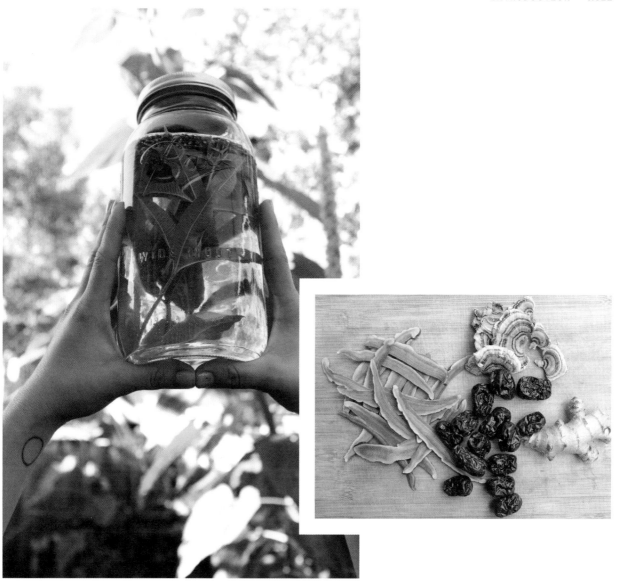

This book is an expression of the elemental practices we use daily and have found the most healing from our study of Western herbalism and Ayurveda. You'll notice that throughout the book we toggle back and forth from the elemental qualities and their Sanskrit names. For us, it's important to use the ancient names while trying to understand what those terms mean in our modern times. Please stick with the terms and concepts that make the most sense to you. We want this to feel tangible and inclusive no matter what your background of healing modalities might be.

Our Practice as Elemental Herbalists

First off, many of you may be asking, "What is an herbalist?" Herbalism is as broad as the practice of medicine. Just because someone practices herbalism doesn't make them a clinical herbalist who sees clients and analyzes lab tests. Our teacher Rosemary Gladstar simply states that herbalists are those who work with the plants. We love this point of view, because it highlights that this path is available to all, regardless of degrees or backgrounds.

With that said, there are certification programs and even degrees in herbalism. Some countries have licensure for herbalists, but the United States doesn't. If you want to see an herbalist under insurance, it's best to seek out a functional doctor who's familiar with herbs or an acupuncturist who is trained in herbalism. Many herbalists, including us, are cautious of state licensure. It could very well make these practices more available, but the standardization and barriers to formalized licensure could drastically limit the ability to incorporate a diversity of plant species (especially hyperlocal varieties) and spiritual practices, and could endanger indigenous and traditional healers. As this practice grows in popularity, please advocate for the initiatives that include and support the diversity of plants and people who are engaged in herbalism.

Herbalists can be farmers, medicine makers, body workers, clinical practitioners, community herbalists, and more—we come in many forms! Our practice as elemental herbalists incorporates elemental theory along with medicinal plants. And as cooks and community herbalists, we rely heavily on kitchen herbalism. We believe that we're more likely to engage in herbal rituals when they feel and taste good. Many argue over the very best format to take a plant, and we always consider this, but our primary concern is that you choose your herbs and stick to a routine of working with them, as this only deepens the relationship you have with your medicine. We find client compliance to be higher and costs to be lower when our clients center their healing around the kitchen.

We offer one-on-one consults online and in person, where we figure out your elemental constitution (*dosha*) and do a health intake. We then work together to come up with herbal-infused recipes and rituals that are best for you, with appropriate dosage and tailored to your energetic makeup. We also teach our ongoing clients how to make

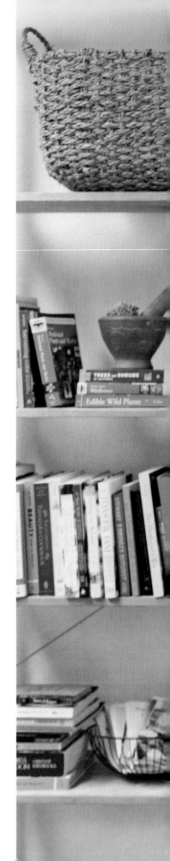

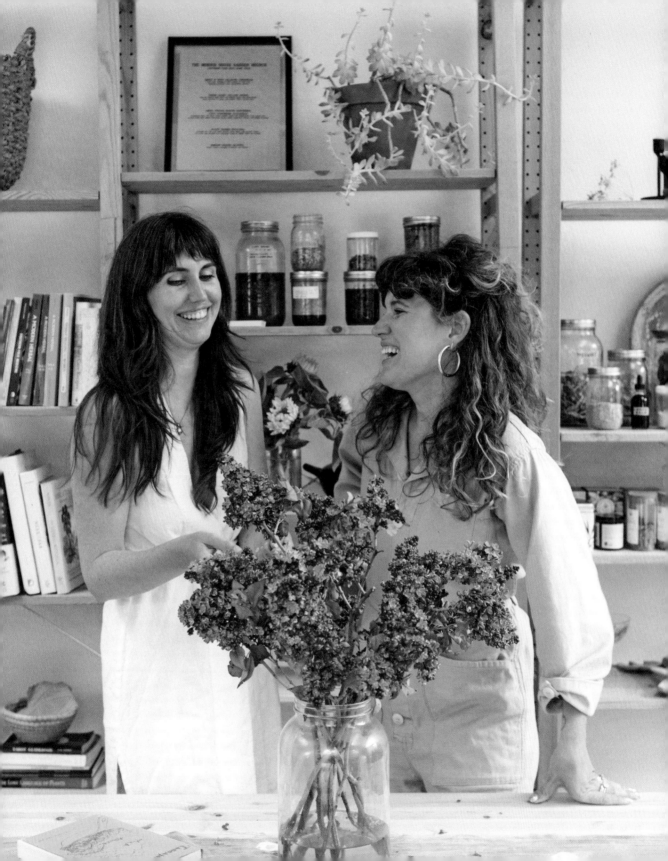

these remedies themselves. If you make it to our studio in Sonoma County, we can even make you a custom tea and spice blend! If you want in-depth training, we offer small workshops and comprehensive online programs centered around elemental and kitchen herbalism (see page 264). These take place in the comfort of your home and can be done at your own pace. We'll teach you how to identify these elemental patterns and how to create seasonal kitchen medicines that work with your routine.

If you're looking to heal something major with the help of someone nearby, we suggest seeking out those who identify as clinical herbalists, those who're locally recommended as herbalists/healers, or Ayurvedic practitioners. In the resources section (page 249), you will find information on the American Herbalist Guild (AHG) and National Ayurvedic Medical Association (NAMA)—both have databases of all of their respective certified practitioners living in the United States. Please note that many healers operate outside of institutions; seeking out community counsel in times of need is always a good idea.

How to Use This Book

When we first began to study herbalism, we were overwhelmed with information. The beautiful and challenging thing about the healing arts in the twenty-first century is that there are so many overlapping systems and access to all kinds of plant medicines. Without an energetic practice, it's difficult to know what herbs and remedies are best.

Herbs are the original drugs. The word *drug* itself originally came from Old French and it means herb or medicine. Herbs are the inspiration and base for many pharmaceutical medicines but they should not be prescribed as such. Herbs don't just treat symptoms, they treat people. For example, there might be hundreds of herbs for anxiety—such as chamomile, skullcap, and passionflower—but knowing which will be most effective for you has to do with your elemental constitution.

In part 1 of this book we dive into elemental theory. We teach you the foundations of healing so that you can apply this layer to any practice, whether it be a self-care ritual or a kitchen remedy. There is also an elemental quiz where you can answer questions based on experiences you've had and then see which elements are most present for you, to help inform which remedies will be the most balancing. In part 2 we cover how to create a kosmic kitchen through developing a foundational knowledge of tastes and herbs, and we give you our favorite tips and tricks for stocking and organizing your space. Part 3 contains all of our herbal recipes and rituals that help us stay balanced through nourishing with the opposite elemental qualities from season to season.

You may notice that this book is not "one size fits all" remedy focused— the idea that you can "take this herb for this ailment"—and we intentionally left this out. We believe there are plenty of herb books out there that help with

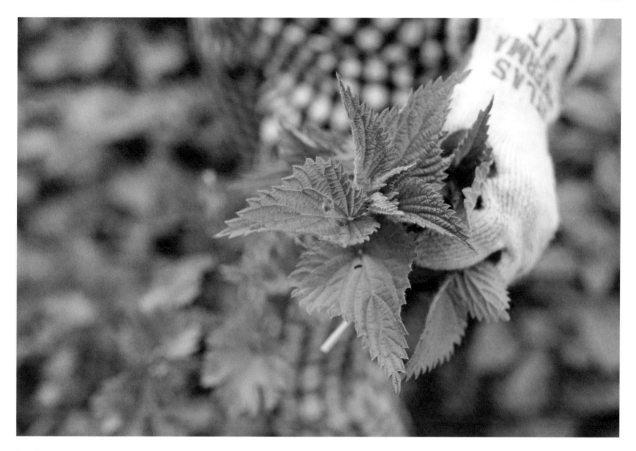

Nettle

specific issues—see our resources section (page 249) for more information on our favorites we refer to regularly. Instead, we wanted to create a fun, inspirational cookbook that encourages you to commit to an everyday herbal practice so that you feel confident creating rituals that work best for you.

We hope you'll use this book as a guide and that you won't take things too literally! We encourage our students to get to know the plants in their own bioregion and use herbs and spices that they already have handy or grow their own. Your wellness practice shouldn't stress you out. We're huge advocates for your everyday herbal practice to be simple and effective, meaning you do you. Just make sure to commit to something, whether that be a daily tea practice, an herbal dressing, or a medicinal breakfast porridge—try to add some herbal goodness in each day.

Ideally, we suggest committing to a full lunar cycle and seeing what comes of it. Use our seasonal charts and elemental lists to stock your kitchen with herbs and foods that will harmonize your elemental constitution. Prep all sauces, dressings, and snacks ahead of time to make life easy. Drink tea and cook a recipe each day, choosing foods and flavors that best suit your elements, and engage in rituals that keep you grounded. If you feel overwhelmed by getting started, simply

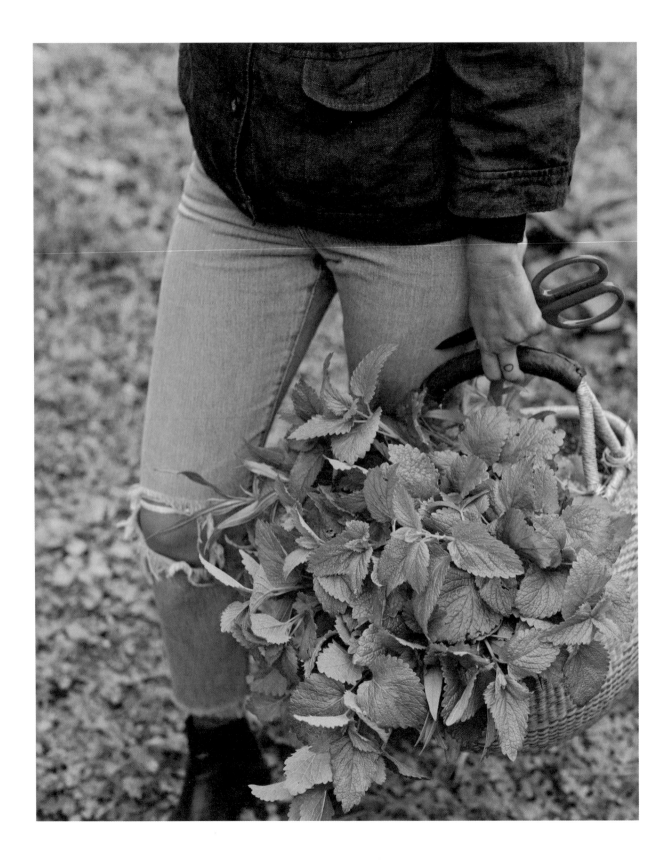

commit to adding in one ritual a day, and gradually you will feel motivated to incorporate more things that make you feel good, and the things worthy of avoiding will be easier to let go of.

Then check in with yourself. Do you feel better emotionally, physically, or both? If you're making progress with what you chose, then keep going. Or perhaps what you've chosen isn't making a positive impact. It's OK to switch things up and rethink your decisions. Just make sure to give enough time to track what has changed, as well as what has not. For chronic issues, it can take a few months to see any major shifts through foods and herbs.

Deep imbalances require deep work and a commitment to protocol, just as you would do with pharmaceutical medications. It's so easy to write off herbs and change courses before you even know what has made a positive effect. Unfortunately, many of us don't understand how powerful herbs are because we haven't been matched up with the right plants and we're not using them consistently at the right dose over time. There is also the issue of herbal quality: not all companies use quality ingredients, so we've created a comprehensive resources section (see page 249).

Of course, when dealing with chronic issues, we believe it's important to work with a clinical herbalist, community herbalist, Ayurvedic practitioner, acupuncturist, or another qualified alternative care provider who can work with doctors, administer lab testing, and tailor your herbal protocol for the specific imbalance you're facing. When we work with folks outside of this system or on a more energetic level, we make sure we share the details we've discovered about our health along the way. All this information helps practitioners to paint a better picture of what's going on. Whether you're in a maintenance period or dealing with major or minor issues, these herbal kitchen practices will always help you feel nourished and supported through the process.

This book has been created with the intention to bring you closer to yourself and the world around you through the practice of elemental herbalism. This way you can have an engaged conversation with your own body and its needs, as well as those who are invested in your healing protocol. Our goal, first and foremost, is for you to be your own best healer and able to advocate for yourself.

Your kitchen will soon begin to transform into a healing sanctuary, where you have collected spices, herbs, and foods that can be mixed and matched to create harmony and balance through the cycles of life. You will develop an herbal literacy and a fundamental understanding of the elements so you can feel confident treating everyday discomforts and supporting the body throughout each season. This place will become your very own kosmic kitchen, where the heart of healing begins.

Sarah Kate

Summer

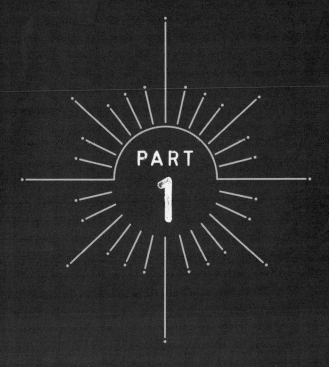

PART

1

"Our five senses serve as the portals between the internal and external realms, as the five great elements of ether, air, fire, water, and earth dance the dance of creation around and within us."

—NAMA INSTITUTE

IT'S ALL ELEMENTAL

Ether   **Air**   **Fire**   **Water**   **Earth**

THE FIVE ELEMENTS—ETHER, AIR, FIRE, WATER, AND EARTH— are the building blocks of life. These elements are all around us and a part of us. All things that exist are made of matter and are elemental by nature. In fact, even our emotions and thoughts hold elemental energies and patterns.

Each element supports one another, and when they work together in harmony they create beautifully balanced inner and outer landscapes, much like we see in the wild. Ether is empty space, or the container in which something can happen. Air is motion or wind in that empty space. Air then enkindles fire, fire changes water (the absence of fire makes ice water or too much fire boils water), water makes the grooves in the earth by creating rivers, streams, lakes, and oceans, and the earth in return allows the foundation for ether to exist. These elemental patterns create a full-circle experience of the seasons and the very existence of our Mother Earth.

When the elemental makeup is imbalanced, the elements can affect each other adversely by expressing as correlated excess and deficiency patterns or illness. These discomforts signal that the elements are no longer working together harmoniously. Understanding elemental theory gives us the tools to recognize these patterns and be our own healer, and to connect more deeply to others and the world around us.

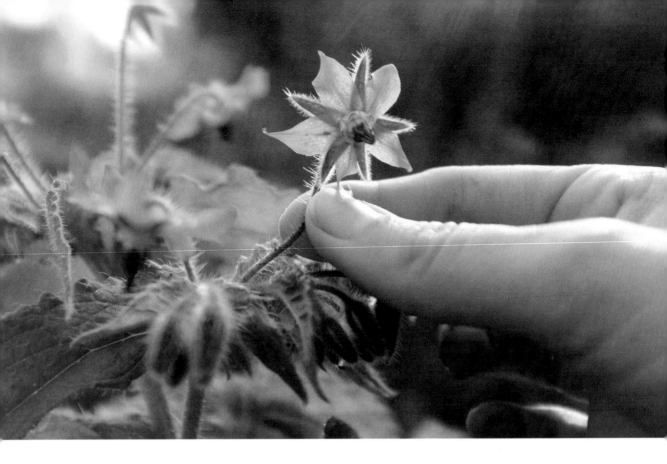

Our ancestors understood the power of the elements—they lived and died by them. Stoves were fed by fire, water required fetching, and the weather could make or break a growing season. Through our practice, we're rediscovering what our ancestors knew all along: we're elemental beings, intricately connected to each other and our ecosystems. And by going deeper, we learn that everyone has a unique makeup, or elemental constitution, as do the plants we use as remedies.

At the root of our unique makeup are the five elements. It's no coincidence that many traditional medicines have woven elemental theory into their practice of healing. Ancient healing traditions and indigenous people worldwide have a long history of using elemental theory to heal and still use these diagnostic practices today. Notably used by (but not limited to) Ayurvedic practitioners, Chinese medicine doctors and acupuncturists, Tibetan medicine doctors, Native American healers, curanderas, shamans, and European herbalists, elemental theory even appears in modern-day chemistry, which was largely influenced by the alchemists.

We've all experienced the elements outside of ourselves. We know what the inviting warmth of a fire feels like on a cold winter's night; how refreshing it is to go for a swim during the heat of summer; the earthy feel and smell of soft, moist dirt beneath our bare feet in spring; and the invigorating chill of a crisp breeze on the first day of autumn. All of these daily experiences with these differ-ent states of matter—the elements—make up the seasons of our lives.

The elements are at work in our body too; they just appear a bit differently. For example, the acids in our digestive system act like fire to help us digest and assimilate nutrients. This heat helps our digestive system create fuel, much like the warmth of a fire does when used for cooking or to create heat for a home. We've also all witnessed the element of water, when in excess it can cause con-gestion. This often shows up when we experience colds and have a stuffy nose. This is why practitioners often suggest avoiding wet and mucus-building foods, such as dairy and sugar, during these times.

Understanding elemental theory helps us navigate the everyday act of balanc-ing. And that choice, to acknowledge the elements and strive for balance, is an essential part of what we like to call "radical wellness." The word *radical* refers to the "root" or "foundation," and it's also a play on words as it nods to an extreme change to the norm. By living in harmony with nature and the elements, we do just that. This connection to nature and the elements helps us stay well and true to ourselves each day. As our teacher DeAnna Batdorff says, "We use Ayurveda and elemental theory all day long, without even knowing we're doing it. When we get too hot, we take our jacket off. When we get thirsty, we drink water. And when we get congested, we choose to blow our nose."

For many of us, with so much of our daily focus and attention turned outward, tuning in to ourselves is a radical act. We aren't always taught how to advocate for ourselves, and we can even feel selfish if we take a few minutes out of our day—or even better, a few hours—for self-care. Being in tune with the body not only gives us a guidepost on a day-to-day level but also enables us to help translate valuable information to practitioners helping us work through and heal illnesses. The goal is to become innately connected to our body, its patterns, and the remedies, so we know exactly what we need to experience relief. We invite you to get radical, cook for yourself, discover the healing powers of plants, and advocate for mind, body, and spirit wellness each day for both yourself and those around you.

Redefining Health Care and Self-Care

Many of us have come on this healing journey out of necessity. Maybe you've experienced ongoing digestive system issues, fatigue, chronic allergies, or other symptoms that are unexplainable and seem untreatable by modern medicine. Per-haps you found a Chinese medicine practitioner, Ayurvedic doctor, or an herbalist or herbal remedy that helped you feel better when other approaches didn't.

Our ecosystems, weather patterns, foods, herbs, and practices all manifest in wildly different ways, but the common thread is the elemental patterns that

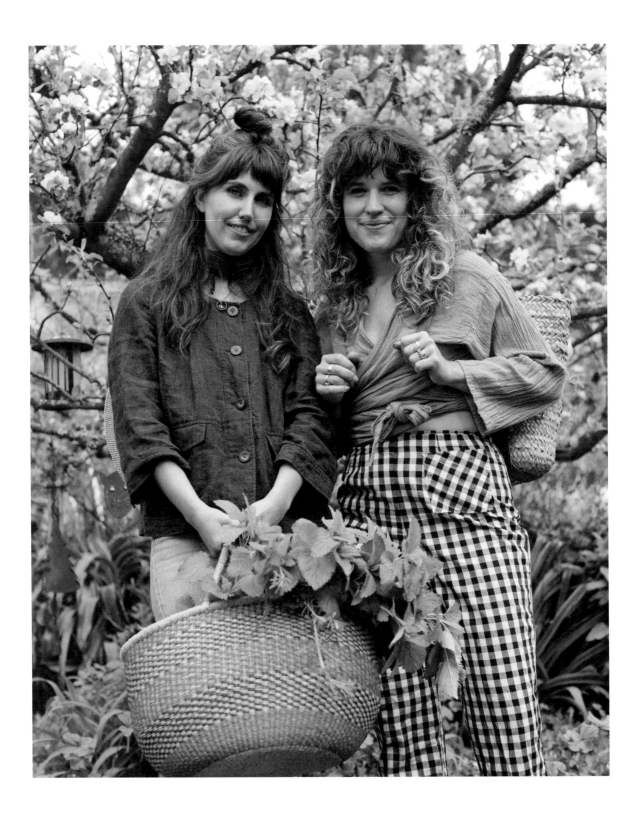

"OUR GREATEST WISH IS THAT YOU FEEL EMPOWERED TO ADVOCATE FOR YOURSELF, GET THE HELP YOU NEED, AND BECOME YOUR OWN BEST HEALER."

come together to create life here on earth. Traditional medicine practices turn to elemental theory to discover underlying patterns and to diagnose and address imbalances rather than just treating symptoms as they arise.

When we merge these traditional healing practices with modern medicine, magic happens. Instead of positioning modern medicine and "alternative" medicine against each other, it's time to create a new all-encompassing medicine tradition. This new pathway to healing will embrace and celebrate the diversity of all healing practices, ecosystems, and people.

We're happy to say that this new paradigm is already happening here in Sonoma County. For some inspiration, the dhyana Center now offers Well Woman Exams and blood work for all. You can get body work with a focus on the lymphatic system, hot compresses and stones, and gua sha massage on the same day you get a clinical Ayurvedic consult, pap smear, and blood work by a nurse practitioner. They're also one of the few Ayurvedic and herbal-focused health centers that accept insurance for specific services. The dhyana Center achieved coverage through the state of California by proving that their clients' quality of life improved and medications were reduced through these services and the elemental education provided during sessions.

We believe that integrating traditional and modern-day medicine is the future and places such as the dhyana Center are paving the way. This unique approach allows for truly holistic protocols that integrate whatever procedures and medications are best for the individual versus merely treating the disease. For one person this may be herbs and talk therapy, and for another it may be pharmaceutical medications combined with body work.

We've both been humbled by our healing journeys, and we firmly believe in using the medicines that are best for you. Get educated on the issues at hand and figure out all of your options. Talk to people in your community and online; you will be surprised by how many people have a shared experience and have gained wisdom through the process. Tune in to your body through meditation and breath work. But the most important thing is to incorporate times of stillness, when you can tap in and feel all the feels. Find a practitioner or center through your network, or by using some of the resources (see page 249) in this book. Know that there is *no* shame in using medications, getting surgery, or even taking herbs!

We're all truly blessed and privileged to live in an era with so many options for healing—the challenge is deciphering which ones to choose. Through this book, you will begin to develop an elemental language that will help you tap into your body to recognize its patterns and what it needs to stay balanced. Our greatest wish is that you feel empowered to advocate for yourself, get the help you need, and become your own best healer.

Elemental Theory through an Ayurvedic Lens

Each healing modality has its own terms or language for talking about the elements, but our background is in the Ayurvedic view of the elements. Our Ayurvedic teacher DeAnna Batdorff strengthened the connection we have to the elements and showed us that elemental theory is accessible and approachable for anyone. Much of our confidence in understanding the elements is owed to her and her years of teaching and service to supporting thousands of people in their healing.

This six-thousand-year-old science teaches how to use herbs from a perspective that goes far beyond a plant's chemical constituents. Though the chemical makeup of plants is important to understanding how plants can help us heal, Ayurveda provides a deeper approach—we're also asked to tune in to our mind, emotions, and spirit as the foundation for wellness. Inherent in the teachings of Ayurveda, and using the elements to guide our healing, is the idea that each individual is capable of self-healing, which just might be the most profound teaching of all.

According to Dr. Vasant Lad and Dr. David Frawley's *The Yoga of Herbs*, the Sanskrit word *Ayurveda* translates to "knowledge of life," which should give you a sense of how vast this science truly is. Unlike modern science, Ayurveda is understood to be a living modality of consciousness channeled into mystic beings known as rishis, or "seers of truth." They discovered the cosmic consciousness that rests in all of creation. Through intensive meditation, daily religious practices, and disciplines, they experienced the truth of being.

The world's oldest sacred texts, the Vedas, encapsulated this wisdom, and from them the eight branches of Ayurveda have been shared throughout the world. They include internal medicine; ears, nose, and throat; toxicology; pediatrics; surgery;

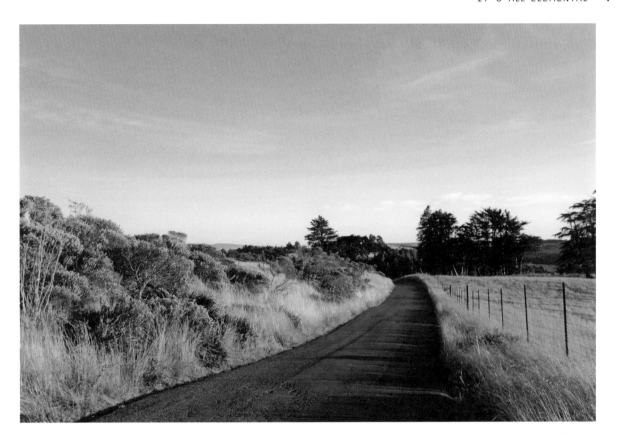

psychiatry; reproductive health; and rejuvenation. In this book we will mostly focus on what Ayurveda would call the branch of *rasayana*, which is all about prevention of illness and increasing vitality and longevity through healthy living.

Over the last decade or so, Ayurveda has had a huge resurgence as people seek a more holistic approach that offers a way to get to the source of their issues or dis-ease rather than just treating the symptoms. People are leaning on Ayurveda and other alternative medicines to answer the questions Western medicine alone cannot. Though many traditional medicines use the elements as their foundation, Ayurveda always resonated strongly with us, and we found elemental theory through this lens to be approachable and user friendly. As modern people working to navigate wellness in a busy and more and more disconnected world, we see this view of the elements to be a powerful ally. We invite you to create your own relationship with the elements in a way that feels best to your unique body and experience.

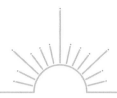

The Five Elements

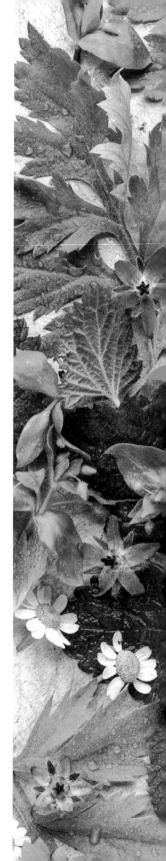

LEARNING TO READ THE LANGUAGE OF THE ELEMENTS can be a powerful tool in creating a healing kitchen. When we first started studying herbs, it was exciting to see how many plants we could use to treat common ailments such as an upset stomach, a mild burn, or a cold. But it can also be overwhelming. We were left wondering, "How do you know which plant to use and when to use it?"

So instead of starting with the herbs, we're beginning with the basics: the language of the elements, understanding their qualities, and how they show up inside and outside of our body. Often the elements are referred to as "energetics," mostly when trying to understand how an herb or remedy will interact with our unique elemental constitution. When we talk about energetics, we're looking at the qualities that are related to a food, herb, environment, and person. Ayurveda refers to elemental constitutions and elemental energies in the body as doshas, and you'll see this explained throughout the book.

For instance, if you hold a cayenne pepper in one hand and a leaf of aloe in the other, you can tell right away that each has different energies. How do you know this? First, you notice that the cayenne pepper is red. This gives you an indication of its warming flavor and the action it will have on your blood or circulatory system. Sometimes when smelling a hot pepper your mouth starts to water, signaling its stimulating potential for the body. Conversely, the aloe leaf feels slightly cool to the touch, it's plump with gel, and has a somewhat bitter smell. These properties indicate aloe's soothing, wet, and cooling nature, and it gives you clues as to what effects its bitter flavor can have on the body.

By tuning in to the power of the elements and their energetic qualities (cold, dry, hot, and wet), you will become aware of their patterns in each season as well as the elemental patterns within yourself. You will begin to tap into yourself on a deeper level. Once you can identify the five elements in your body and their qualities, you can ask yourself, "Am I running cold? Dry? Hot? Wet?" It will become easy to decide what meals to eat, herbs to take, and rituals to perform so you can stay well and thrive each day.

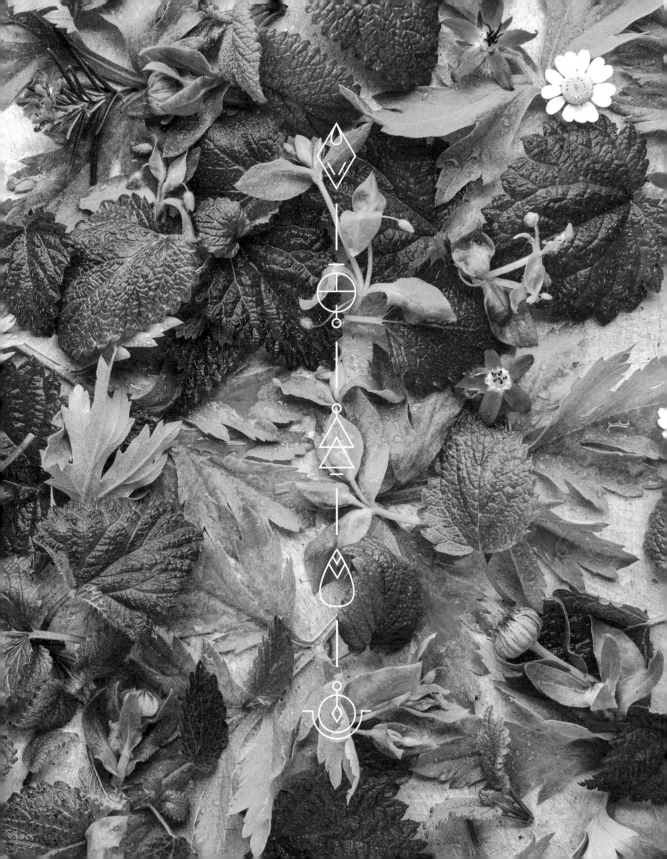

ETHER

ATTRIBUTES: Cold, clear, light, soft, subtle

Ether is empty space, or the container for life. It's referred to first because it's the subtlest of the elements and, in a way, the foundation for the elements to follow. Have you ever heard someone say "You're out in the ethers"? That's a way you might tell someone they seem as if they're mentally off in space. Ether is also associated with the quality of being cold. In the body, ether (or empty space) can be found in the mouth, nose, hollow organs of the digestive and respiratory systems, tissues, and even cells. It's also related to the energies of freedom, love, and expansion.

AIR

ATTRIBUTES: Dry, light, mobile, rough, subtle

Air is the movement of ether. We can't see air, but we feel its effects. Too much air or wind can be drying to the body and disorienting to the mind. In the body, the element of air is the movement or pulsation and contraction of our hollow organs, and it's responsible for gaseous exchange in the small intestine, colon, heart, and lungs. As it's an action that evolves from ether's empty space, it becomes the force behind movements of all kinds.

FIRE

ATTRIBUTES: Hot, penetrating, sharp, spreading

We need enough air to make fire or create heat. Fire is associated with fueling the body, regulating body temperature, and absorbing nutrients. Often you'll hear fire referred to as digestive power, meaning how well the body can digest and assimilate food. Because of this, it's associated with the digestive organs: the stomach, liver, gallbladder, and spleen. Fire is essentially light, which is necessary for us to see, perceive, and create intelligence.

WATER

ATTRIBUTES: Fluid, liquid, oily, slimy, soft

Heat from the sun melts the snow high in the mountains to form our freshwater streams, rivers, and lakes. This liquid element is essential to all life. The human body and the planet are made up primarily of water, about 70 percent each, and water creates the flow of life. Water is associated with the digestive secretions, saliva, mucus membranes, lymphatic fluid, cardiovascular system, kidneys, and pericardium (the membrane that surrounds the heart). It's cleansing and cooling by nature, and it promotes cohesion and flow.

EARTH

ATTRIBUTES: Dense, heavy, slow, thick, static

Earth is the culmination of all of the elements manifested into physical form. All the elements start with ether, but all elements are ultimately represented in earth. The grounded and solid nature of earth is the basis of all life—from the human body to the plants and minerals that make up our environment. Earth is considered the structure of the body and is associated with all tissues, organs, glands; and it's the manifestation of all the elements combined. The earth element provides a foundation or structure for all things.

Tuning In to the Seasons

Each season has dominant qualities that determine our experiences, the foods we eat, the herbs we use, and the wellness practices we lean on. The qualities of the elements (cold, dry, hot, wet) are our cues for each season.

In Ayurveda, there are three main seasonal energies that correlate with the three doshas—*vata, pitta, kapha*. In this book we've elaborated on how the doshas and elements overlap with our Western perspective of the four seasons. However, if the seasons feel differently in your ecosystem or don't fit into a four-season model, simply apply the practice of opposites to find balance to nourish and stay well. When it's hot you can lean into cooling remedies, and when it's dry you can incorporate moistening and building rituals, and vice versa. Simply connect with your own body and the season to discover the present qualities and incorporate the opposites to remedy any imbalance.

Let's take a deeper look at how the elements appear throughout the four seasons. (Also see the charts for each season in part 3.) Having more awareness of the elements at play will help us know where we're out of balance and how to come back into ourselves, but first we must know how to feel and identify them. You'll also notice that no element is singular; instead, they all cycle back to and build on one another. This is the truest form of a holistic system.

SEASONS AND THEIR QUALITIES

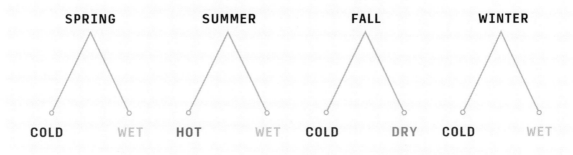

SPRING		SUMMER		FALL		WINTER	
COLD	WET	HOT	WET	COLD	DRY	COLD	WET

This is just one general example of how the elements can come to life seasonally. Depending on your ecosystem, the dominant qualities may be different from season to season.

SEASON: FALL THROUGH EARLY WINTER

ELEMENTS: Ether and air

QUALITIES: Cold and dry

DOSHA: Vata

As the leaves of the trees begin to turn golden and fall to the earth, we enter the season of fall. This time is marked with cooler, drier days. Usually the drop in temperature and lack of moisture in the air create a feeling of dryness in our environment and our bodies. Sweet root vegetables and squashes are collected during this harvest season; this taste naturally helps build and moisten our bodies so they stay nourished through the colder times of year. During this time, you will want to focus on getting grounded and staying nourished, as it's easy to want to move and constantly change course with all the cold, airy energy.

Ether and air present themselves so we can turn our attention to the organs most affected by these qualities. Our hollow organs responsible for gaseous exchange in the body—such as the small intestine, colon, lungs, and heart—need extra attention as they're easily affected by cold and dryness.

Perhaps during the autumn months you've come down with a cold, experienced digestive issues such as constipation or gas, felt more anxious than usual, had stiff joints, or noticed your hands or feet were cold. These are common symptoms of the elements of fall showing up in the body.

SEASON: LATE WINTER THROUGH SPRING

ELEMENTS: Water and earth

QUALITIES: Cold and wet

DOSHA: Kapha

When rain or snow starts to fall and the trees are bare, we know we've entered into the darkest time of year: winter. Fall and winter are similar in that they're both cold, but winter, with its precipitation, brings moisture. During this season, we want to slow down, even if our lives don't easily allow it. Wet and cold in combination feel heavy, slow, and even sluggish if not in balance. You may have experienced respiratory issues, feelings of fatigue or lethargy, and depression or other emotional upsets during winter. It's important to incorporate warming and stimulating plants and rituals so you stay invigorated through these dark and damp times.

The cool days and rain typically continue as we head into springtime. Budding blossoms paint the gray landscape with their pastel hues, signaling a change in season. During this period, wild greens and herbs start popping up, providing us with fresh bitter flavors to help our bodies gently cleanse and release any heaviness we've accumulated from winter.

Focusing on the organs that are associated with the cold and wet qualities will bring strength during the gray days of winter and spring. Supporting the bladder, kidneys, pericardium, and lymphatic and circulatory systems will help maintain balance.

SEASON: SUMMER THROUGH EARLY FALL

ELEMENTS: Fire and water

QUALITIES: Hot and wet

DOSHA: Pitta

At the end of the wet season, we're greeted by longer, hot and sunny days. Depending on where you live, summer can be hot and dry or hot and wet. Where we grew up in Florida, the summer was hot but daily thunderstorms created a lush subtropical, junglelike ecosystem. Now, living in Northern California, the summer is hot and dry, often with scorched hillsides from wildfires. Simply adjust to remedy with the opposites, depending on if your summer is wet or dry. Either way, it's important to incorporate cooling rituals that promote flow.

During the summer we can tend to feel more inflamed and aggravated, experience seasonal allergies, and have hotter digestion that can lean toward diarrhea. Focusing on the hot and wet organs of digestion and assimilation will help quell these uncomfortable experiences. The stomach, liver, gallbladder, and spleen are the organs that need the most support this time of year.

———————◇———————

Now that you've gotten a better sense of the elements, their qualities and seasonal expressions, and a bit about Ayurveda's view on them, we'll show you how the four qualities—cold, dry, hot, wet—create the five elements and the elemental constitutions. This is the basis of using elemental theory as a daily tool. You'll

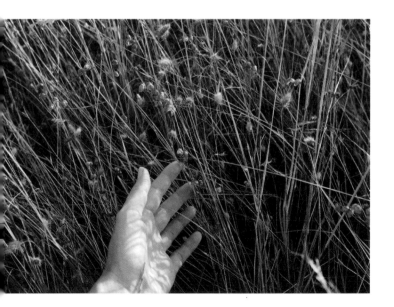

begin to see the physical, emotional, and spiritual connections the elements play in your life. This is why we're so passionate about sharing this work with you.

It's really a way to start communicating with your body and understanding what your body is trying to communicate back to you. It puts the power back in your hands, allowing you to tap into what you already know, letting you decipher and honor your gut feelings. Learning to read the elements will make choosing foods, remedies, and practices feel true to you and your overall state of well-being and balance.

Our Bodies, Our Elements

Each of us has a unique combination of the five elements within us. Our elements are passed down from generation to generation—just think about the similarities you share with your parents. Perhaps you have a similar hair color as your mother, or maybe you share a sense of humor with your father. We're born with all the elements, but usually a combination of two will be dominant. The ancient seers recognized these patterns, or doshas, of how the elements expressed themselves in different people, and then they predicted how the patterns would inform physical, mental, and emotional states.

We're taught by modern society that there is an idealized body, temperament, or pace to structure our lives around. The real truth is that each body is unique and has its own set of strengths and weaknesses. Knowing this allows us to quiet the noise of having to fit a mold that doesn't feel right and find a sense of self-acceptance.

The elements can empower you to tune in to yourself each day and ask, "What do I need?" Instead of having to reinvent the wheel of your wellness routine, the elements can provide a foundation to come back to when you feel off or out of balance. If you start to think about these elemental patterns as archetypes that support you in finding balance, the doshas will feel more like guides rather than symptoms of imbalance. The elements are malleable and never static; they're in a constant ebb and flow from moment to moment. Instead of feeling overwhelmed by this, you can let go and realize that we're always in a state of balancing. Balancing is a dance, not a destination.

ELEMENTAL QUIZ

This quiz will help you start to see the patterns of the elements within your body and how they express themselves. If you've ever seen an Ayurvedic or Chinese medicine practitioner, many are trained in the ancient art of pulse reading as one of the first diagnostic tools to see what's going on in the body, mind, and spirit. Reading the pulse helps to determine not only acute and chronic symptoms but also your innate nature being expressed through the qualities of the elements. This is one of the traditional ways that practitioners can determine your specific elemental imbalances and constitutions. This book doesn't focus on pulse reading, but it is a great diagnostic tool, so we recommend that you see practitioners in person who have tools such as pulse, face, tongue, and/or energetic diagnostic skills to help give you a more in-depth picture of the elements at play within you and how they're expressing themselves.

This simple quiz will introduce you to your body and its elemental patterns, and it will give you a foundational awareness from which you can begin your kosmic kitchen practice. When taking the quiz, think of it as a loose guide to help

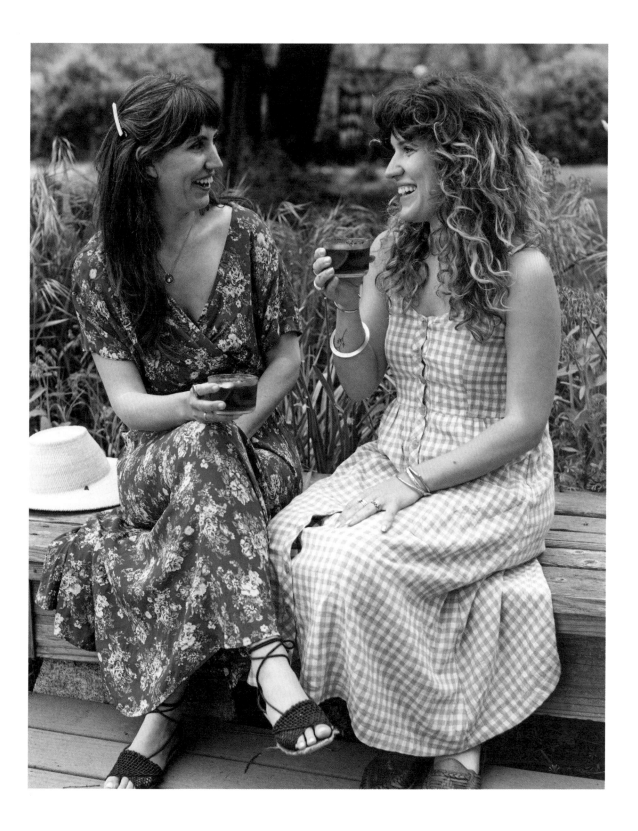

you start to notice the patterns you hold in day-to-day life. You should take the quiz two ways. First, take the quiz through the lens of your childhood experience. This will give you a picture of the elements that make up your foundation, or what is known in Ayurveda as *prakruti*, or your birth constitution. Then, take the quiz thinking about how you're feeling right now, or how you have been feeling over the past few months, to help reveal your current state, known as *vikruti*.

To take the quiz, read the question and choose one letter (a, b, or c) that intuitively feels the most like you. Simply tally up the letters when you're done and see which two letters you have the most of. This will indicate your dominant elemental patterns. In the following section we'll explain the elements and the doshas that they create. Ultimately, this quiz is meant to inspire you to take a closer look at your day-to-day patterning that can serve as a cue to watch as your body makes shifts throughout different seasons, environments, ages, and experiences. We encourage you to work with an herbalist versed in elemental theory or an Ayurvedic practitioner to learn more about your elemental constitution. We offer online and in-person elemental herbalism consultations for those looking to deepen their connection to the elements and their herbalism practice. See our resources section (page 249) for more information on practitioners.

How would you describe your physical structure?

a. Petite

b. Muscular

c. Curvy

Would you describe your skin as being more:

a. Dry and rough

b. Red, sensitive, or prone to inflammation and rashes

c. Cool and oily

Does your body feel:

a. Boney

b. Toned

c. Thick

Does your hair tend to be:

a. Dry and frizzy

b. Straight and prone to gray and hair loss

c. Thick and oily

When you speak, does your voice tend to be:

a. Quiet and reserved

b. Loud and direct

c. Melodic and comforting

Does your body temperature run:

a. Cold; it's hard to break a sweat

b. Hot; you sweat easily

c. Cold and wet—you're cold but also a bit sweaty at times

Does your breath tend to be:

a. Shallow

b. Restrained

c. Labored

Do your bowel movements tend to be:

a. Constipated and pellet-like

b. Loose and acidic

c. Gassy and mucous prone

Do you like to eat foods or have cravings for foods that are:

a. ☐ Dry and crunchy

b. ☐ Spicy, acidic, and oily

c. ☐ Dense and sweet

Concerning sleep patterns, do you find it:

a. ☐ Difficult to fall asleep and your sleep is easily disrupted

b. ☐ Easy to fall asleep when you want to

c. ☐ Easy to fall asleep and hard to wake up

What are you most prone to?

a. ☐ Colds and flus

b. ☐ Allergies and inflammation

c. ☐ Sinus congestion and fatigue

What best describes your appetite?

a. ☐ You tend toward low blood sugar and feeling hungry often

b. ☐ You can go a long time without eating but you still have stamina

c. ☐ You have a low appetite in the morning, tend to eat a little throughout the day, then indulge in rich or sweet foods in the evening

What ecosystems do you feel most comfortable in?

a. ☐ Warm, wet, and humid, such as a tropical climate

b. ☐ Cold and dry, such as a high desert climate

c. ☐ Warm and dry, such as a Mediterranean climate

When under stress do you tend to:

a. ☐ Worry and want to escape, or become irritated easily

b. ☐ Overwork and tend toward anger or frustration

c. ☐ Become depressed, shut down, and in the muck

When working in a group do you tend to be:

a. ☐ The idea person, super creative

b. ☐ The leader, putting ideas into action

c. ☐ The supportive role, making sure things flow harmoniously

Your friends tend to come to you for:

a. ☐ Creative inspiration

b. ☐ Analyzing and problem solving

c. ☐ A shoulder to cry on

Things that come easily to you are:

a. ☐ Discipline, routines, and spiritual concepts

b. ☐ Intellectual ideas, focused activities, and responsibility

c. ☐ Nurturing, supporting and loving others, being grounded

When in conflict you tend to be:

a. ☐ Fearful and put up a lot of boundaries

b. ☐ Direct and easy to anger

c. ☐ Defensive and stubborn

What weather aggravates you?

a. ☐ Windy, dry, and cold, like a cold fall breeze

b. ☐ Hot, wet, and humid, like summer showers

c. ☐ Cold and wet, like rain and fog

Your emotional state when out of balance tends to be:

a. ☐ Fearful and anxious

b. ☐ Angry and resentful

c. ☐ Grieving and depressed

A: _____   B: _____   C: _____

Tally your results for each letter and mark the two letters that you have the most of. These indicate your primary and secondary doshas. It's possible that you will have a nearly equal balance of all three doshas. Learn more on how to interpret your results on the following page.

ELEMENTAL QUIZ RESULTS

A	B	C
You're mostly ether and air elements with cold and dry qualities, known as the vata dosha	You're mostly fire and water elements with hot and wet qualities, known as the pitta dosha	You're mostly earth and water elements with cold and wet qualities, known as the kapha dosha

HOW TO INTERPRET THE RESULTS

This quiz is simply meant as a guidepost. You can use the results to better understand the elemental patterns that you're most prone to and adjust specific nourishment and rituals accordingly. As you dive further into this book and your studies, you will get a better handle on your elemental constitution. We highly suggest seeing a practitioner, so you can get all your specific questions answered. This is especially helpful when you're addressing ongoing health issues versus a maintenance phase.

Please note that the lens with which you take this quiz will also determine the results. If you think of how you were as a child while taking it, it will yield results that are closer to who you are innately, that is, your birth constitution. As we grow older and encounter sickness and trauma, it's possible that our imbalances sway our experiences and bodily manifestations of the elements. Where we are now, in this moment, is known in Ayurveda as vikruti—lifestyle imbalances that show us which elements need our attention. That's why it's so important that even with natural and traditional medicines you seek the help of a professional to guide your way in times of illness.

To keep it simple, it's best to tune in to how you're feeling at the moment and reflect the cues of the season when deciding on the best herbs and foods for nourishment. *Return to those two questions—Am I running hot or cold? Am I feeling dry or wet? Then nourish and restore balance with the opposite qualities.*

As you interpret these results and look at them through the lens of your birth constitution, or prakruti, you will likely have a primary or dominant dosha and a secondary dosha. In other words, the letter you have the most of reveals your dominant elemental pattern; the next highest is your secondary elemental pattern. If you're more or less equal in your results, it's possible that you're tridoshic, though that is less common. Remember that we can relate to all energetics and doshas, because we have experienced each of them at one time or another.

UNDERSTANDING THE PRIMARY AND SECONDARY DOSHAS

When choosing remedies for balancing the doshas, which we'll go over in the next section, let the season be your guide. From there, look at which qualities of the

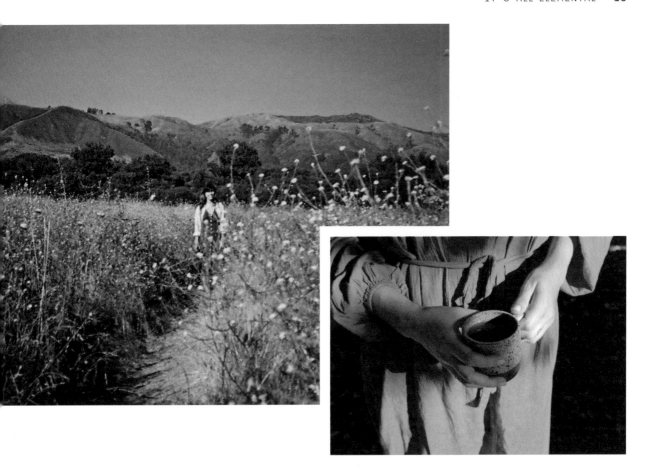

season are the most present—cold, dry, hot, and/or wet—and where your own constitutional qualities overlap. When there are shared qualities, you can easily create an excess.

As always, you will want to create balance by using remedies with the opposite qualities. In the case of the season being in energetic opposition to your primary dosha, such as fall (vata season) with pitta dosha, you will by nature be less challenged by the season as you're innately creating a balance. You may wish to nurture your secondary dosha instead, if it feels aggravated by the season. For example, if you're a primary pitta dosha with a vata secondary dosha, you'll want to focus on balancing different qualities throughout the changing seasons. During the summer months (pitta season), you will need to focus on balancing your pitta, the hot and wet qualities that can become exacerbated during the warmest months of the year. So, you'll be looking for foods and remedies that are the opposite—cooling, fresh, more alkaline, and soothing to any inflammation that might occur.

Then as you head into fall (vata season), you'll find your secondary vata dosha needs more attention during the dry, windy, cool days. So, you'll want to focus on remedies that are warming and moistening—soups, stews, and warm milky teas, for example—to help soothe frayed nerves and help the body ground during the transition into fall.

As a pitta-vata heading into cold winter (kapha season), you're still keeping an eye on the qualities of cold, wet, and dry, as these qualities are dominant in the season and represented within your primary and secondary doshas. Again, you are focusing on remedies that are warming and soothing in nature, but being mindful to not overdo hot spices, acidic foods or beverages, or overindulge in sweets around the holidays that can aggravate your pitta dominant nature, even when it's cold outside.

Please note that depending on your ecosystem, the seasons may have different qualities, so it's important to integrate the meaning behind these phrases. If your winter is actually cold and dry versus cold and wet, simply strike a balance by using the opposite qualities. At the end of the day, we should be in tune with our bodies and our environments from moment to moment.

COMBINATIONS OF AYURVEDIC DOSHAS AND THEIR QUALITIES

VP: VATA (ETHER/AIR)—PITTA (FIRE/WATER)   →   QUALITIES OF COLD/DRY AND HOT/WET

VK: VATA (ETHER/AIR)—KAPHA (WATER/EARTH)   →   QUALITIES OF COLD/DRY AND COLD/WET

PV: PITTA (FIRE/WATER)—VATA (ETHER/AIR)   →   QUALITIES OF HOT/WET AND COLD/DRY

PK: PITTA (FIRE/WATER)—KAPHA (WATER/EARTH)   →   QUALITIES OF HOT/WET AND COLD/WET

KV: KAPHA (WATER/EARTH)—VATA (ETHER/AIR)   →   QUALITIES OF COLD/WET AND COLD/DRY

KP: KAPHA (WATER/EARTH)—PITTA (FIRE/WATER)   →   QUALITIES OF COLD/WET AND HOT/WET

VPK: VATA (ETHER/AIR)—PITTA (FIRE/WATER)— KAPHA (WATER/EARTH), A.K.A. TRIDOSHIC   →   QUALITIES OF COLD/DRY HOT/WET, AND COLD/WET

The Four Qualities: Cold, Dry, Hot, and Wet

COLD QUALITIES

Cold as a quality is expressed as the depressed tissue state in traditional Western herbalism, the vata or kapha doshas in Ayurvedic medicine, or yang deficiency in Chinese medicine. Cold is the quality of ether, or empty space—the ethereal realm, or the container in which matter and energy are held. Cold on a physical level feels contracting or stagnant in the body, especially when in excess. Emotionally or energetically, cold can feel heavy, removed, or unkind—likely you've had the experience of someone being rude or "cold" to you. Seasonally, cold is represented by the fall and winter seasons, the times we feel naturally inclined to support our systems with the opposite quality, warmth.

Most often we experience cold in our bodies through the circulatory system. We might have cold hands or cold feet, the physical sensation of cold in our extremities. Cold can manifest in an imbalance of digestive secretions or acids, meaning we don't have enough fire to break down and assimilate our food. Emotionally, it can be difficult to self-motivate when we're cold, which affects our zest for life and leads to fatigue.

Cold needs to be supported with warming remedies, mostly in the form of liquids and heavier nourishing foods; see the fall and winter recipe sections on pages 182 and 216 for examples. Leaning on flavors that are sweet, pungent, or sour helps combat cold and support healthy circulation. Anytime we're in a cold environment or season, it's important to dress warmly to create a buffer from the temperature. A daily ritual of oiling the body, or Abhyanga (page 214), creates a warm and soothing barrier that not only helps to instantly nourish the nervous system by hydrating the largest organ (our skin) but also creates a layer of protection around the body. Taking warm baths and creating soothing environments help to calm feelings of fear and anxiety that cold can exacerbate.

DRY QUALITIES

Dry as a quality is expressed as the atrophied tissue state in traditional Western herbalism, the vata dosha in Ayurvedic medicine, or yin deficiency in Chinese medicine. The quality of dry often goes hand in hand with cold. Dry is expressed through the element air, the element of movement and rapid change. Physically, this quality arises as dry hair, nails, skin, or eyes. Digestively, when we're dry we experience constipation or hard, small, compact stool. When we feel dry in our bodies or environments it can cause feelings of anxiety, indecision, or excessive mental chatter (overthinking). It can feel as though our nerves are fried and we feel raw to the world around us, which leads to irritation.

Seasonally, dry mostly shows up in the late summer and fall seasons. There can be a sense of feeling scattered—we're easily swept up in distraction during this time of year. It's not just the season that can perpetuate the feeling of dryness in our bodies. Technology and constant stimuli from the modern world add to the depletion of the kidneys and adrenal glands, causing us to feel as if we must always be on, much like our devices.

Taking time for soothing rituals that are hydrating and nourishing, such as Herbal Steams (page 146) or warm baths, will help counterbalance the feeling of dryness. That goes for our foods and herbs as well. We need moistening, cooked foods that are sweet and salty, such as miso soups, broths, and porridges. Making sure we're giving our bodies a daily oil massage is key to combating dryness, along with taking breaks from technology to be outside, engaging the elements. More moistening remedies and rituals can be found in our fall recipe section (page 182).

HOT QUALITIES

Hot as a quality is expressed as the excited tissue state in traditional Western herbalism, the pitta dosha in Ayurvedic medicine, or yang excess in Chinese medicine. Hot is related to the element of fire, which embodies the spark that has the power to transform. As a reminder, the fire is birthed from ether (empty space) and the air elements—all elements flow in succession and riff off one another. Hot on a physical level has a warm and spreading quality, which, when out of balance, can lead to all kinds of inflammation. Emotionally or energetically, hot can feel fiery, impulsive, and angry. Seasonally, hot is represented by the abundant summer season. To stay balanced through a hot time or season, it's best to support with the opposite quality, cold.

Some time or another we've all experienced heat in the body, notably in the digestive system. An excess of the hot quality often creates acidity in the gut, which can lead to acid reflux, oily stool, or even diarrhea—anyone who's eaten too much spice can relate! It also manifests physically in excess through inflammatory responses, as your body is signaling you to slow down and cool off. Inflammation or heat can be expressed as chronic immune issues, allergies, skin issues, headaches, and even body pain. Emotionally, the hot quality can make you hot headed, which is an old phrase for someone who has a quick temper. This excessive heat, which is often coupled with a go-getter attitude, can ultimately lead to burnout. All hot fires need fuel to keep burning.

Hot needs to be supported with cooling remedies. Look to foods with bitter, astringent, or sweet flavors to calm excess heat and inflammation. Think of things that are cooling, fresh, alkaline, and raw—see our summer section for recipe ideas (page 148). Lean into the green by incorporating sprouts, salad greens, and fresh pesto. Infuse cooling and calming herbs, such as lemon balm and chamomile, and the ones found on page 34 under the pitta list. Try meditating, yin yoga, or taking long walks to restore a sense of calm. You may also wish to incorporate a daily abhyanga practice, with cooling oils such as coconut and essential oils such as lavender and chamomile—see page 179 for more rituals for the hot quality.

WET QUALITIES

Wet as a quality is often expressed as the damp tissue state in traditional Western herbalism, pitta and kapha doshas in Ayurvedic medicine, or yin excess in Chinese medicine. Cold is related to the element of water, which comes after the transformation of (or lack of) fire. It embodies flow and cohesion. Wet on a physical level, when out of balance, can feel slimy, oozy, or like congestion. Emotionally or energetically, wet can feel sluggish, stagnant, depressed, "stuck in the mud," or it can even embody excess (too much water can create a flood). Seasonally, wet comes up in seasons with rain, fog, snow—whenever that is for your ecosystem. This is often during snowy winters, spring showers, or even humid summers.

The quality of wet, which is responsible for our lymphatic system, is actually a part of our immune system. You may experience the wet quality when your body creates excess mucus during a cold and your lymph nodes are swollen. Wet can also manifest as congestion or stagnation in the gut or body, such as mucus in the

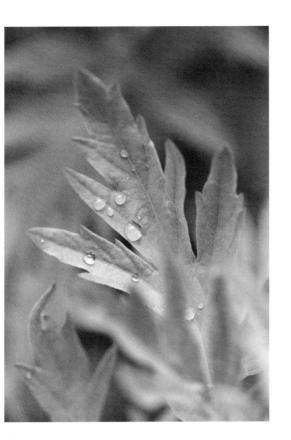

digestive tract. When wet combines with hot, it looks more like excess sweating, diarrhea, or oozy infections. Too much nourishment, fluid, or water creates mud in nature and mucus, swelling, and puffiness in the body. This is the body speaking up, trying to cleanse itself from the excess of the wet quality.

Wet needs to regain balance through incorporating drying remedies, mostly things that are astringent, bitter, pungent, and sour. If it's wet and cold, we look to kapha remedies that are warming and drying. Look to page 116 for recipes and rituals for the kapha season and page 37 for your food and herb list. During this time, you'll lean into lots of veggies, bitter greens, uplifting herbs such as tulsi, and you'll avoid dairy (which builds mucus). If it's wet and warm, you'll need drying and cooling. Look to page 148 for recipes and rituals for the pitta season and page 32 for your food and herb list. In this case, you will need more raw and alkaline foods, uplifting and bitter herbs such as lavender and lemon balm, and food seasoned with lots of warming spices. Try incorporating Dry Brushing (page 145) into your daily ritual to activate the lymphatic system, move stagnant energy, and promote a healthy immune system through proper flow.

Mugwort

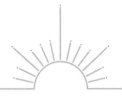

The Elemental Archetypes

NATURALLY, THE COMBINATION OF THE ELEMENTS creates their own archetypes or constitutional patterning. Since our minds learn well and can take in information easily by association, building a framework for each dosha will create a relatable picture of just how the elements express themselves through our physical bodies, temperaments, and imbalances. It's likely that when reading through the archetypes, you'll find similarities to not only yourself but those you're close to as well. As you begin to understand our natural human inclinations, you will see yourself and those around you more clearly and find an opening to acceptance and compassion. We're all on a journey and dropping the judgment toward ourselves and others can have a profound impact in the healing process.

No dosha is better than another. Each has its own set of strengths and weaknesses. The more we learn about our dosha, the better we will become at identifying how to stay more even keel, rather than swinging from one extreme to the next. Again, keep in mind your primary and secondary doshas. You'll want to give more attention to supporting the dosha that relates to the season you are in currently. For example, if it's springtime (kapha season) and your dominant dosha is vata (cold and dry) but your secondary dosha is kapha (wet and cold), you'll want to use remedies that help balance kapha, since it will be more aggravated by the cold and wet environment.

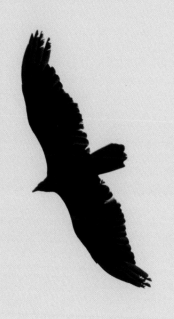

Ether ◈ and Air ⊕
Archetype: Vata

The expression of the vata dosha is the constitution of the subtle body—ether and air. Ether and air are known to be constantly changing or mobile in nature. People who are predominantly vata tend to be dreamers, creatives, and spiritually guided, living from a place of intuition rather than logic, much like artistic Aquarians of the zodiac. They pick up on energetics or vibrations easily, and if they're grounded in themselves, this can be a powerful tool in decision-making. They're quick to learn and love to share ideas and connect with others.

Having a quiet, calm space suits vata constitutions best, as they're highly aware of their environments and too much outer stimuli can be overwhelming. They need alone time to meditate, pursue creative projects, and ultimately tap into their intuition. Vatas are drawn toward mysticism, philosophy, and spiritual or monastic life. It can be a challenge for them to commit to a routine, but consistent healthy rituals will be their biggest ally for showing up authentically in the world. Being in nature is their ultimate medicine; it brings them into their body so they can feel grounded while tapping into cosmic energies.

Physically, vatas experience more cold and dry qualities than others. This shows up in Western herbalism as depression and atrophied tissue states. They often have cold hands and feet and dry skin, hair, or nails. Structurally, they either tend to be on the petite side or tall, and they're slender and have somewhat irregular features. They don't have as much digestive fire—that is, the ability to break down and assimilate food—so they can have drier digestion that leads to constipation. Being less rooted in the stability of the earth makes vata people susceptible to anxiety, fear, worry, and indecision. Vata is also the quality that is most easily thrown off balance, especially with our constant use of technology. Incessantly checking our devices creates a sense of having to be alert or on all the time. It depletes the adrenal glands and strains the nervous system. You've probably experienced that feeling of your nerves being fried after a full day of staring at the computer screen.

Cold and dry qualities can be soothed by warming and nourishing remedies. Enjoying soups and stews or cooked foods helps create more fire in the digestive system and requires less moisture to break down food into nutrients. Cold and dry types do best with warm beverages and should avoid cold, carbonated, or caffeinated drinks. Supporting the organs ruled by the ether and air qualities is important for creating balance. The hollow organs that allow gaseous exchange such as the lungs, heart, small intestine, and colon will be the first indications of imbalance. The bones and nerves are also part of the ether and air elements and should be nourished by mineral-rich, hydrating, and soothing remedies.

Remedies are always the opposite of what we're experiencing. So, if we feel scattered, ungrounded, and empty, we need to focus on foods, herbs, and

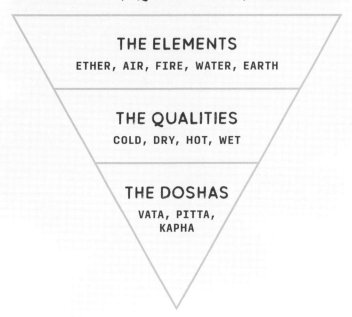

ELEMENTS, QUALITIES, DOSHAS

THE ELEMENTS
ETHER, AIR, FIRE, WATER, EARTH

THE QUALITIES
COLD, DRY, HOT, WET

THE DOSHAS
VATA, PITTA,
KAPHA

practices that are nutritive and build us up, ground us back into our bodies, and create a soothing place to relax into. Coming home from a long day to a comfortable environment with soothing music, putting on soft clothing, and enjoying a warm bowl of soup is a great routine for vatas to help relieve anxiety and foster a sense of calm.

A VATA IN BALANCE

I am aware of the subtle energies around me. When I am grounded in myself, I can tap into my intuition for guidance and know that it will never lead me astray. My greatest strength is being able to dance between the spiritual and material planes to bring insight and new ideas to the world. By being warm and nourished in my body, I'm able to express divine creativity in my work, personal life, and relationships. I feel held by the earth and look to nature for support when I feel ungrounded, anxious, or fearful. My life feels full when I am in my body, in touch with my feelings, and able to show up for others with warmth and acceptance.

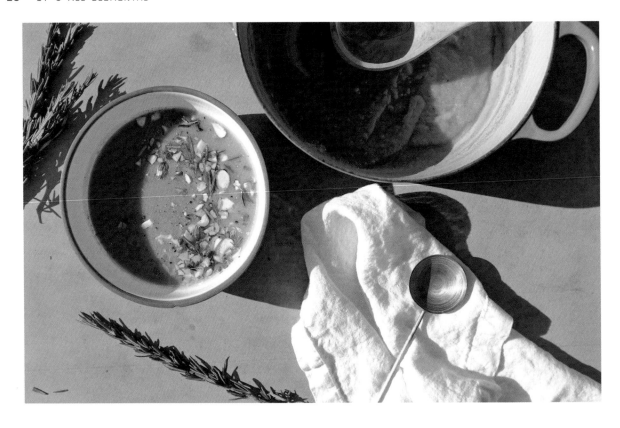

FOODS AND REMEDIES THAT BALANCE COLD AND DRY | VATA

This is a list of foods commonly found at grocery stores and farmers markets that are beneficial for the vata dosha. Don't consider this list comprehensive; we encourage you to use your taste buds as a guide and notice the sensations you feel to determine the qualities of food you eat. This is especially helpful when traveling to new places and experiencing new produce.

TASTES: Sweet, salty, sour, pungent

FOODS: Focus on meals that are mostly wet and cooked, such as soups, stews, milky teas, and broths. Grounding foods such as roots and vegetables will create a sense of fullness and contentment when experiencing cold and dry in the body.

VEGETABLES: Asparagus, avocados, beets, bok choy, carrots, leeks, mustard greens, okra, onions, pumpkin, rutabaga, squash, sweet potatoes, zucchini

FRUITS: Apples (cooked), apricots, bananas, berries, cantaloupe, cherries, coconut, dates, grapefruit, grapes, kiwi, lemons, limes, mangoes, melons, oranges, papaya, peaches, pineapple, plums, rhubarb, tamarind, tangerines

LEGUMES: Fava beans, kidney beans, red lentils, mung beans, soybeans (tofu, tempeh, or miso)

GRAINS: Amaranth, oats, quinoa, rice, teff, whole wheat

ANIMAL PROTEINS: Beef, chicken, duck, eggs, fish, lamb

OILS AND FATS: Almond oil, avocado oil, coconut oil, dairy (preferably raw) in moderation, ghee, olive oil, safflower oil, sesame oil, sunflower oil

NUTS AND SEEDS: Almonds, brazil nuts, cashews, coconut, macadamia nuts, pecans, pine nuts, pistachios, pumpkin seeds, sesame seeds, sunflower seeds, walnuts

SUGARS: Brown sugar (unrefined), date sugar, honey (raw), maple syrup

SPICES: Basil, cardamom, celery seed, chilies (in small amounts), cilantro, cinnamon, clove, coriander, cumin, curry leaf, fenugreek, ginger, lemongrass, rosemary, sage, salt (ocean or river), sumac, tarragon, turmeric

MEDICINAL HERBS FOR COLD AND DRY | VATA

The herbs listed here are categorized to give you a sense of how they can support different body systems. Because it's ruled by ether and air, the vata dosha will be more easily susceptible to imbalances with the nervous system. So, focusing on herbs that support a feeling of warmth, nourishment, and calm will be a major key to maintaining a balanced sense of self.

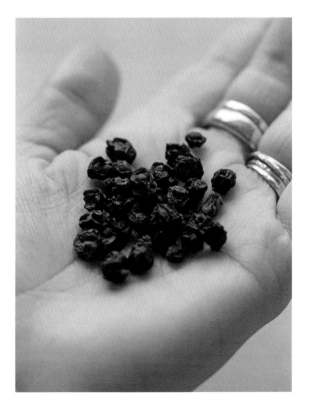

While many herbs fall under these categories, we've included "warming and moistening" digestive system herbs and a whole category of herbs to promote proper circulation. Some of these herbs may only have one of these two balancing qualities, meaning they aren't always both warming and moistening. Remember that you can always add in warming or moistening herbs, foods, or spices to balance an herbal formula or meal.

CALMING NERVOUS SYSTEM HERBS: These herbs help support the nerves acutely under stress, but they're best used over time to restore nervous system vitality. In herbalism we call these herbs "nervines." Most of these herbs fall under the warming or moistening category, while others can be combined with herbs or spices that are more warming to offset their cooling nature.

Chamomile, lemon balm, milky oat, rose, skullcap, tulsi, valerian

WARMING AND MOISTENING DIGESTIVE SYSTEM HERBS: Mostly spices, these herbs are wonderful to add to foods for their flavors and digestive support.

Cardamom seeds, cinnamon, fennel, ginger, licorice, marshmallow

Schisandra

NOURISHING AND RESTORATIVE HERBS: These herbs are great to include in everyday formulas to help balance feelings of cold or dryness.

Ashwagandha, lemon balm, licorice, milky oats, shatavari

IMMUNE SYSTEM HERBS: Including these herbs in your routine will add more warmth, promote circulation, and boost the immune system in order to help the body ward off acute colds and flu-like symptoms. Astragalus root should be used prior to getting sick as a preventative medicine.

Astragalus, elderberry, elderflower, garlic, ginger, reishi, turmeric

SKIN, LYMPH, AND LIVER HERBS: Use these herbs to soothe the skin and provide gentle support for the lymph and liver. Dandelion and burdock are on the cooling and bitter side, so make sure to add warming herbs or spices when using regularly.

Burdock, calendula, dandelion, tulsi, milk thistle, turmeric

CIRCULATORY SYSTEMS HERBS: Mostly spices, these warming herbs support healthy circulation for cold and dry imbalances.

Cayenne, cinnamon, ginger, hawthorn berries, rosemary, sage, schisandra

ADAPTOGENS FOR VATA: These are adaptogens that have more warming or moistening energetics helpful for balancing vata.

Ashwagandha, eleuthero, licorice, maca, schisandra, shatavari

FLAVORS AND FOODS TO AVOID

Bitter, astringent, cold, and raw foods will aggravate the feelings of cold and dry. Pickled foods, vinegars, strong ferments, ice cream, and caffeine are too cooling and astringent and will put out your digestive fire. When vata people are stressed or anxious, it's easy to reach for dry, crunchy snack foods such as popcorn or chips, which will only exacerbate cold and dry qualities. To reduce anxiety and create warmth and a sense of stability, eat three full meals that are warming, naturally sweet, and protein rich.

SELF-CARE PRACTICES

Warming and soothing rituals should be anchors for any vata's self-care regime to help balance the elements of cold and dry. Gentle movement that connects you to your breath will not only help calm anxious tendencies in the mind but also bring you back into your body and ultimately connect you to your intuition.

Try some of these practices: Warming Winter Salt Scrub (page 244), warm baths, daily Abhyanga (page 214), warming footbaths, warming Herbal Steams (page 146), swabbing sesame oil in nose and ears to soothe dryness, breath work, light exercise and movement.

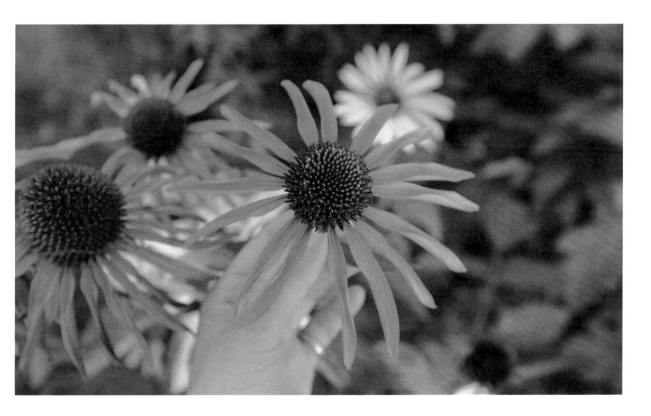

Fire 🔥 and Water 💧
Archetype: Pitta

When fire and water meet, they create a force to be reckoned with. In Ayurveda, this combination of elements is the foundation of the pitta dosha. People with this constitution are fiery go-getters with a high intellect who often do well in the spotlight or in leadership roles. They're often active, with plenty of energy and a passionate lust for life, much like Leos of the zodiac. They're the kind of people who can fit in anywhere. Whether leading a meeting of CEOs or hanging out at the local dive bar, they have no problem relating to others, in many different contexts, and finding common ground.

Physically, pittas often have big, curly (frequently red) hair and strong muscular features, and they love to flaunt their excitement for life by wearing vibrant clothing or unique pieces of adornment. They're often active and big on sportsmanship, and they can often easily build muscle. They greatly benefit from rigorous exercise to help them blow off steam and excess. They do well with meditation and breath work at the start and end of the day to center and calm their fiery nature.

It's important for this fire sign to cool it with spicy and acidic foods, so nightshades such as peppers, tomatoes, and eggplants should be consumed in moderation. Fried and oily foods are often their Achilles' heel and are best avoided. Instead, they should focus on nourishment that is cooling, calming, and drying. If their fire is running too hot, they may need to hydrate with more moistening foods and herbs.

The pitta constitution governs digestion, which includes the liver and gallbladder. When the fire and water elements are out of whack, the liver and gallbladder are often the first systems to fall prey to illness. So, pittas can be prone to acidic digestive issues, high blood pressure, heat-related headaches, skin issues, rashes, and infections. On the emotional side, hotheadedness, irritability, impatience, defensiveness, and sharpness can emerge. These imbalances are often a result of too much fire, which can arise from working too hard, forgetting to eat, or living in excess.

Pittas thrive when their fire is burning slow and steady and fueling their passions. Out-of-balance fires produce anger, irritability, overwhelm, rashes, inflammation, and infections. When in balance, pittas are emotionally in tune, steady, and passionate.

PITTA IN BALANCE

I live a life of passion and flow. I am powerful and resilient, and I know that grounding rituals nourish me and my life's purpose. I am a leader, and I know that everyone with whom I create serves a role and purpose that is just as important as my spark. I know that strength can also be fed by vulnerability. I am open to looking at myself honestly and communicating directly with others. My life is vibrant, and I embody passion by loving myself first so that I may share my gifts with the world.

FOODS AND REMEDIES THAT BALANCE HOT AND WET | PITTA

The pitta constitution thrives on cooling, fresh, and alkaline foods. Flavors that work best include sweet, bitter, and astringent tastes, all of which help quell excess fire. Think raw or steamed greens and other foods that are fresh and non-aggravating. This constitution also does well with daily tonics that are mineral rich, such as nettle, and calming herbs, such as chamomile and lavender, to keep stress at bay. Adaptogenic herbs will help reduce stress by nourishing and tonifying the endocrine system and bolstering the immune system. Such herbs can be wonderful allies for pittas who tend to work long hours and need extra herbal help to support their passions and avoid burnout.

TASTES: Sweet, bitter, astringent

FOODS: Focus on meals that are mostly raw, cooling, fresh, and alkaline, especially in warmer weather. Brothy, light soups and fresh foods such as raw vegetables and vegetable juices, salads, collard or lettuce wraps will provide minerals, nutrients, and energy without stoking your fire.

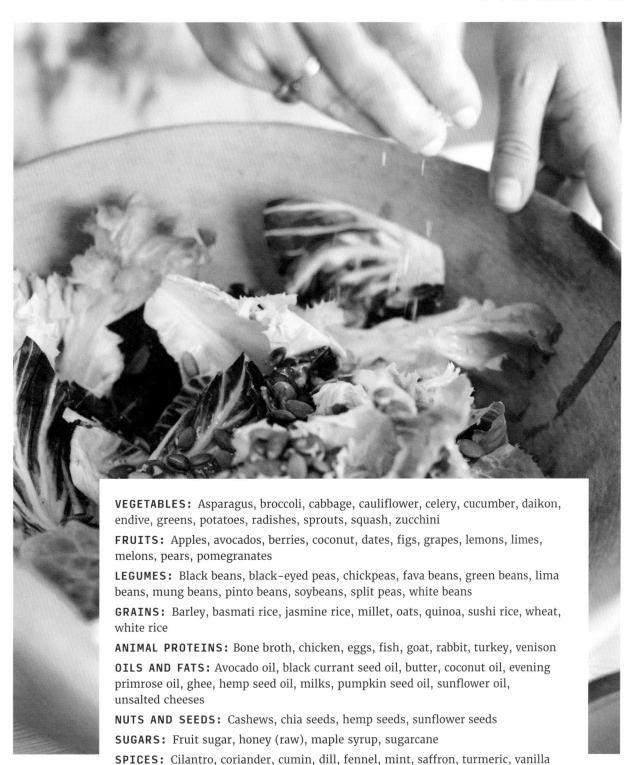

VEGETABLES: Asparagus, broccoli, cabbage, cauliflower, celery, cucumber, daikon, endive, greens, potatoes, radishes, sprouts, squash, zucchini

FRUITS: Apples, avocados, berries, coconut, dates, figs, grapes, lemons, limes, melons, pears, pomegranates

LEGUMES: Black beans, black-eyed peas, chickpeas, fava beans, green beans, lima beans, mung beans, pinto beans, soybeans, split peas, white beans

GRAINS: Barley, basmati rice, jasmine rice, millet, oats, quinoa, sushi rice, wheat, white rice

ANIMAL PROTEINS: Bone broth, chicken, eggs, fish, goat, rabbit, turkey, venison

OILS AND FATS: Avocado oil, black currant seed oil, butter, coconut oil, evening primrose oil, ghee, hemp seed oil, milks, pumpkin seed oil, sunflower oil, unsalted cheeses

NUTS AND SEEDS: Cashews, chia seeds, hemp seeds, sunflower seeds

SUGARS: Fruit sugar, honey (raw), maple syrup, sugarcane

SPICES: Cilantro, coriander, cumin, dill, fennel, mint, saffron, turmeric, vanilla

MEDICINAL HERBS FOR HOT AND WET | PITTA

The herbs listed here are categorized to give you a sense of how they can support different body systems. Because it's ruled by fire and water, the pitta dosha will be most susceptible to general inflammation issues and digestive distress. This is why we have listed "soothing" digestive system herbs and "cooling" restorative herbs.

While many herbs fall under these categories, we've included the ones we've worked with and have cooling or drying qualities that are helpful for pitta imbalances, seasons, and doshas. Some of these herbs may only have one of these two balancing qualities, meaning they aren't always both cooling and drying. Remember that you can always add in cooling or drying herbs, foods, or spices to balance an herbal formula or meal.

CALMING NERVOUS SYSTEM HERBS: These herbs help support the nerves acutely under stress, but they're best used over time to restore nervous system vitality. In herbalism we call these herbs nervines. Most of these herbs are fairly neutral but lean more toward the cooling and drying qualities.

Catnip, chamomile, hops, lavender, lemon balm, milky oats, passionflower, skullcap

SOOTHING DIGESTIVE SYSTEM HERBS: These herbs are cooling, calming, and relatively neutral. It's best to avoid marshmallow if you're feeling too much of the wet quality. These are great plant allies for those with a hot (often dry) and inflamed gut lining and need help restoring it.

Calendula, chamomile, coriander, cumin, fennel, lavender, lemon balm, marshmallow, peppermint, plantain

COOLING AND RESTORATIVE HERBS: These vitamin-rich green herbs are great to add in during times when you're hot and feel as though you need replenishment.

Alfalfa, aloe, chickweed, cleavers, horsetail, nettle

IMMUNE AND RESPIRATORY SYSTEM HERBS: Infuse these plants into your life when you're feeling run down. Marshmallow root and slippery elm are great for those moments when you're feeling hot and dry or have a sore throat. Elderflower and yarrow are cooling diaphoretics—they help the body "sweat it out" in the early phases of a cold. The others are fairly neutral but will help boost your immune system when you need it most.

Echinacea, elderberry, elderflower, marshmallow, mullein, yarrow

SKIN, LYMPH, AND LIVER HERBS: These plants, called alteratives in herbalism, are cooling, neutral to drying. They promote healthy skin (acne, rashes, and skin issues commonly affect pittas) through supporting the systems of elimination, especially the lymphatic system and liver function.

Aloe, burdock, calendula, chickweed, chicory, cleavers, dandelion, nettle, plantain, red clover, rose

ADAPTOGENS FOR PITTA: These adaptogens are cooling and will help balance and rejuvenate the pitta dosha when used consistently over time. Tulsi and schisandra are both warming, but they will do well to reduce the wet qualities of pitta when paired with cooling herbs.

Astragalus, licorice, reishi, schisandra, shatavari, tulsi

FLAVORS AND FOODS TO AVOID

Avoid oily foods and spicy, salty, and pungent tastes as well as table salt, fried foods, and stimulants such as chocolate and coffee. It's also best not to consume too many nightshades such as eggplant, peppers, and tomatoes in excess, as they're acidic. Nuts, especially peanut butter, can be aggravating to this constitution because of their oily nature—try consuming seeds instead.

SELF-CARE PRACTICES

Cooling and cleansing rituals should be anchors for any pitta's self-care regime to help balance the elements of hot and wet. Activities that are intentional, slow, or easy will not only help you ease the desire to always be working or doing but also bring you back to a place of calm and relaxed effort.

Try some of these practices: Abhyanga (page 214) with cooling oils such as coconut or sunflower oil, breath work, calming teas, cold plunges, meditation, swimming, walks, or yin yoga.

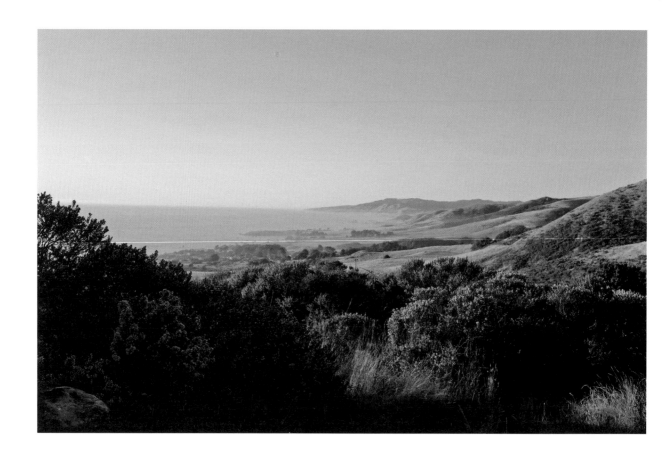

Earth 🜨 and Water 🜄
Archetype: Kapha

The earth and water elements flow together to create life. Fluids needs a container—a vein, vessel, or river—to carry their essential nutrients, and their container is earth. In nature, these elements, which make up the kapha dosha, show up as green and blue, and when in harmony they create nourishment. This archetype is the mother, the essence of comfort, much like Cancer on the zodiac. These people crave stability, harmony, and pleasure for both themselves and the people around them. In Chinese medicine this would be a yin archetype, and in traditional Western herbalism it's considered a damp or relaxed tissue state.

Kaphas usually have a full, curvy body structure with plump and hydrated skin. They often have thick, oily, and luscious hair, and large eyes. They also often have a strong, hearty build and a radiant glow.

Imbalanced kaphas can overdo it in the name of a cause. They're loving human-itarians who live to support others—sometimes at the expense of their own health. This can come into play by working too many hours, taking on the sole supportive role in a family, or even repressing their needs. Kaphas are also prone to sluggishness.

Flow is in their nature, but when earth and water elements don't move, they create mud. Sluggish kaphas can have trouble with follow-through, exercising, and overindulging, and they can be sensitive. Physically they're prone to bloating, swelling, constipation, and excess mucus.

When in flow, this watery archetype is home to people you can count on: caregivers or those who provide nourishment and love to others. While slow, they're also steady; they will get things done in harmony and without drama. They're loving beings who truly embody the essence of the earth mother—grounded, rooted, and powerful.

KAPHA IN BALANCE

I live my life for love, but I love myself first and foremost. I nourish myself fully so that I may nourish my community. I am active, steady, and stable. I know that movement and flow keep me grounded and in my body. I am a nurturer, and I know that the magic of nourishment is dependent on the dose. I provide endless love, but I do not enable myself or others. I am wise beyond my years, and I know that the longevity of my energy and effort is important to my whole being. My life is full of love and community, and I embody the essence of the earth by living in harmonious flow.

FOODS AND REMEDIES THAT BALANCE COLD AND WET | KAPHA

Kaphas thrive off of nourishment that comes in the right dose. Too much or too little can wreck their day. They need to feel supported in order to do their nurturing work in the world, but too much grounding can make them sluggish and fatigued. It's important to incorporate raw or lightly cooked foods, no matter the season. Lots of vegetables are key, while carbohydrates and sugars should be eaten in moderation. Dairy should mostly be avoided, as this can aggravate the wet quality. Add a bit of invigorating spices to all foods. Also try incorporating uplifting herbs such as peppermint, lemon balm, and tulsi for everyday tonics.

TASTES: Sour, pungent, bitter

FOODS: Focus on foods that are warming, drying, and cleansing, and incorporate lots of raw and fresh vegetables. Lean on fresh salads, raw vegetable juices, and light invigorating meals. Make sure to season food with lots of spices to increase enzymatic actions and digestive fire.

VEGETABLES: Arugula, asparagus, bok choy, broccoli, brussels sprouts, burdock, cabbage, carrots, cauliflower, celery, chard, collard greens, corn, daikon, dandelion, eggplant, endive, garlic, jicama, kale, kohlrabi, leeks, lettuce, mustard greens (and greens in general), onions, parsnips, peppers, radishes, spinach, sprouts

FRUITS: Apples, apricots, berries, cherries, citrus, figs, grapes, lemons, limes, peaches, pears, persimmons, pomegranates

LEGUMES: Black beans, black-eyed peas, chickpeas, lentils, lima beans, navy beans, pinto beans, soybeans, split peas, white beans

GRAINS: Amaranth, barley, buckwheat, corn, millet, quinoa, rye, wild rice

ANIMAL PROTEINS: Buffalo, eggs, fish, white poultry

OILS AND FATS: Black currant seed oil, borage oil, fish oil, flax seed oil, ghee, goat dairy, olive oil, pumpkin seed oil, sunflower oil

NUTS AND SEEDS: Poppy seeds, pumpkin seeds, sesame seeds, sunflower seeds

SUGARS: Honey (raw) and all sugars in moderation

SPICES: Basil, bay leaf, caraway, cardamom, cinnamon, cloves, coriander, cumin, curry, garlic, ginger, marjoram, mustard, nutmeg, onions, orange peel, oregano, paprika, peppers, rosemary, saffron, sage, star anise, sumac, tarragon, thyme, turmeric

MEDICINAL HERBS FOR COLD AND WET | KAPHA

The herbs listed here are categorized to give you a sense of how they can support different body systems. The kapha dosha, ruled by earth and water, will be more susceptible to a sluggish lymphatic system, congestion, and melancholy. This is why we have listed "uplifting" herbs and "stimulating" digestive system herbs.

While many herbs fall under these categories, we've included the ones that we've worked with and have warming and drying qualities that are helpful for kapha imbalances, seasons, and doshas. Some of these herbs may only have one of these two qualities, meaning they aren't always both warming and drying. Remember that you can always add in warming or drying herbs, foods, or spices to balance an herbal formula or meal.

CALMING AND UPLIFTING NERVOUS SYSTEM HERBS: These herbs are pungent and a balancing taste for kapha, but many of them are primarily cooling. Cold needs warming, so be sure to prepare with warming herbs such as ginger and cinnamon. The uplifting nervines are important to kaphas who, when out of balance, can become overwhelmed and down.

Catnip, chamomile, hops, lavender, lemon balm, passionflower, rosemary, skullcap

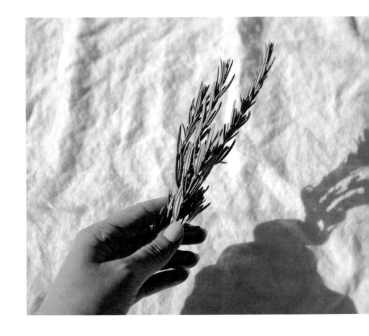

STIMULATING DIGESTIVE SYSTEM HERBS: Cold and wet qualities often need warming and stimulating plants to promote circulation and proper digestive system function, as excess kapha can breed sluggishness and even constipation. These plants are warming and pungent, which both promote circulation.

Anise, cardamom, dandelion, ginger, hibiscus, lavender, lemon balm, peppermint

NOURISHING AND RESTORATIVE HERBS: These herbs—all neutral to cooling— have pungent and cleansing qualities. Pair with warming foods or herbs if you feel you need more stimulation. These plants come up in the spring, and they're often incorporated into herbal foods during this cold and wet season for postwinter replenishment.

Alfalfa, aloe, dandelion, nettle, plantain

IMMUNE AND RESPIRATORY SYSTEM HERBS: Kaphas tend to become congested and sick when their immune system is weak, due to the cold and wet qualities. We incorporate warming, drying, and pungent herbs to stimulate flow and release congestion. Many of these herbs are great in steams or teas when you're feeling stuffy and runny.

Echinacea, elderberry, elderflower, elecampane, garlic, ginger, eucalyptus, oregano, sage, thyme, yarrow

SKIN, LYMPH, AND LIVER HERBS: These pungent herbs stimulate lymph flow. Pair with ginger, cinnamon, or other warming spices to heat up a formula or dish.

Calendula, chicory, cleavers, dandelion, plantain, red clover, rose

ADAPTOGENS FOR KAPHA: These adaptogens work over time to restore vitality of the whole body. They help the body become more resilient and capable of dealing with internal and external stressors. These adaptogens are all warming, which is ideal to strike a balance against kapha's cold quality.

Ashwagandha, eleuthero, maca, schisandra, tulsi

FLAVORS AND FOODS TO AVOID

Sweet, wet, cold, and dense foods. Avoid refined and processed carbohydrates, sugars, and dense meals. Avoid overeating and overindulging. It's best not to consume too much dairy, as this can create more of the wet and cold qualities in the body. Think about cleansing, raw foods instead, and warming spices to create balance.

SELF-CARE PRACTICES

Warming and cleansing rituals should be anchors for any kapha's self-care regime to help balance the elements of cold and wet. Invigorating movement that connects you to your breath will not only help create a sense of warmth and move stagnation but also bring you back into your body and ultimately connect you to your energy.

Try some of these practices: Abhyanga (with warming oils, see page 214), baths (with warming and invigorating herbs), breath work, cardio, cupping, Dry Brushing (page 145), heated yoga, running, walking (especially after meals).

Putting It All Together and Creating a Seasonal Practice

Now that you've learned about the doshas, their qualities, and the remedies that will help create a sense of balance, you might be thinking, "How do I navigate this seasonally?" For instance, if you took the Elemental Quiz and found that your elements seem to be on the opposite ends of the spectrums, such as hot and cold (pitta/vata) or wet and dry (kapha/vata), you're not alone. The thread that pulls all four qualities together is the season you're currently in. That is always the focus when looking for balancing remedies, since the qualities of the season in your environment will have the greatest effect on your body.

Let's say your primary dosha is vata, so the qualities you experience the most are cold and dry. One the other hand, your secondary dosha is pitta, meaning you also have qualities that are hot and wet. How do you navigate these seemingly opposite doshic qualities? Again, let's look to the season. During the cooler months of the year, your focus is on the vata qualities of cold and dry because these qualities will be more easily out of balance. You'll want to nourish with warming, moistening, and grounding foods and beverages to offset the cooling nature of your environment. Same goes for the herbs you take and your self-care rituals. Think warming spices such as cinnamon, cardamom, and ginger—flavors we naturally gravitate toward during the winter holidays. Our ancestors who created these winter traditions already knew the warming effect these comforting flavors have on the body. Focus on medicinal herbs that build the nervous system and warm the circulatory system such as ashwagandha, tulsi, and hawthorn. Hot baths, Herbal Steams (page 146), and deep breathing will help offset the restricted and contracted nature of the cooler months and help you stay grounded in your body.

As the season begins to shift from cool to warm, you'll want to think about balancing the hot and wet qualities of your constitution. If you live in an area that is hot and dry, choose remedies and practices that are cooling, cleansing, and moistening. Focus on fresh foods and herbs to help cool and refresh your body during the long hot days of summer and help balance any inflammation, irritation, or allergies that are common this time of year. Being in a relaxing natural environment, swimming in cool fresh water, making time to rest and not overwork are wonderful rituals to stay in balance this time of year.

When the warmer months begin to wane and the cooler season approaches, lean on the practices that support warmth in the body, once again. Remember

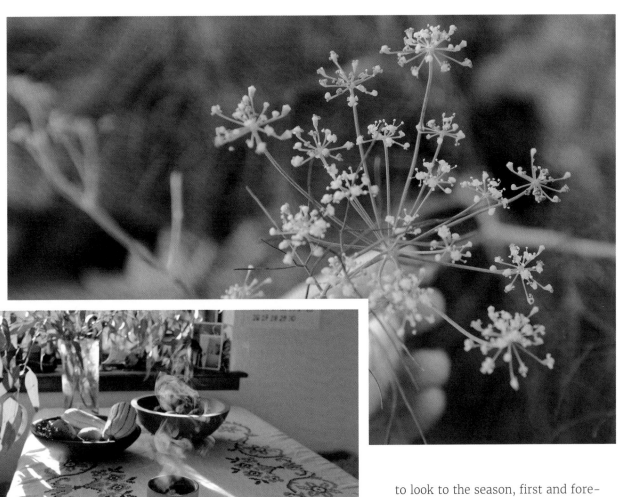

to look to the season, first and fore-most, for guidance, then check in with your own elemental makeup to see which qualities—cold, dry, hot, or wet—are the most similar at this time. That will be the quickest way to know which doshic qualities to prioritize for balancing during that season.

Now that you're connecting with your elements, remedies, and rituals, let's get into the kitchen so you can make this whole balancing thing a part of your everyday routine. In the next section, we'll show you how we use common herbs found in grocery stores, Western herbs, and Ayurvedic and Chinese herbs, along with nourishing foods to create a kosmic kitchen. Instead of feeling overwhelmed by cooking each day, approach healing by making your kitchen feel like a sacred space, filling it with your favorite healing remedies. You'll find that creating a nourishing meal can come together in no time when you already have your staples in place and have done a little preparation beforehand.

PART

2

"*Learn to listen when a plant speaks, to speak to the plant as to another human being, and to look upon it as one's teacher.*"

—DR. VASANT LAD & DR. DAVID FRAWLEY

CREATING A KOSMIC KITCHEN

FOR HERBALISTS, THE KITCHEN IS MORE THAN JUST A PLACE to cook. It's a place where all the elements—ether, air, fire, water, and earth—meet to make medicine. We see our kosmic kitchen as both an apothecary and an altar. It's where we dry herbs, burn incense, and create adaptogenic ghee under the glow of the moon. Some days we chant over our medicines in ancient Sanskrit, and other times we chop herbs to the rhythm of Erykah Badu. Every medicine maker is going to have their own playlists, plants, and rituals. But at the root of creating and maintaining a kosmic kitchen is honoring the sacred: our bodies, our spirits, and the plants. Once this container is created, magic happens.

We experience magic as the connection we feel to ourselves, our loved ones, and the Earth. There's a groundedness from being a part of the elemental processes at play. When rooted, we're able to tune in to our internal guides—our intuition—and find the clarity of what is truly nourishing. Putting ourselves first and taking time to care for our own needs can feel like a radical act in a world filled with distractions and a never-ending to-do list. Whether this nourishment comes in the form of enjoying a meal, taking a warm bath, or going on a walk, the right remedy is there if we slow down and listen.

To reduce expense and stress, we focus on plants, ingredients, and practices that are more easily accessible, so you can focus on the magic of healing. We believe the best medicines are the ones you'll actually take, and the ones you'll have fun making. This part of the book is meant to guide you in creating your own kosmic kitchen. We're going to teach you how to create sacred space, stock and organize your apothecary, and feel empowered to choose the right remedies and recipes for you.

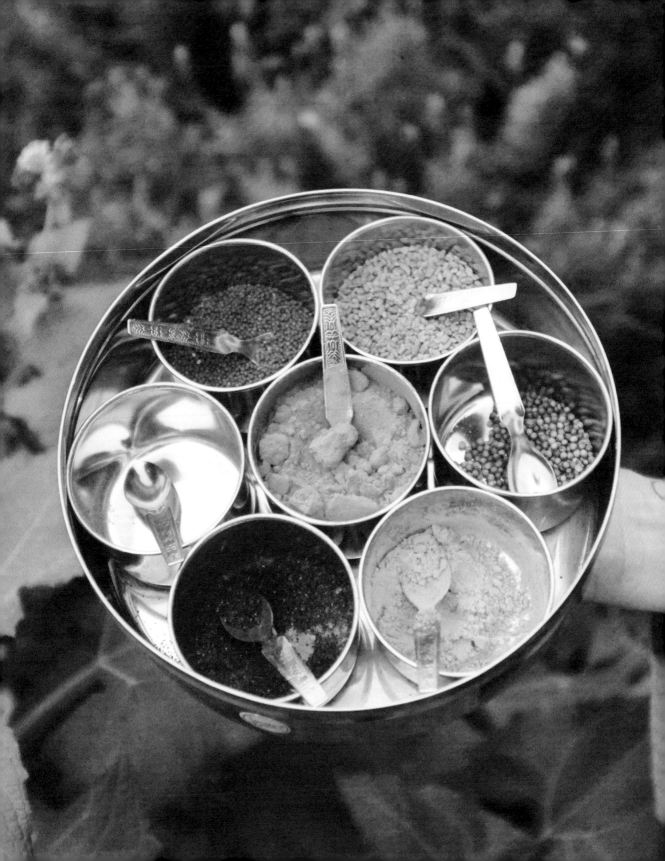

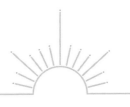

The Elements of Taste

USING THE SIX TASTES HELPS US RECOGNIZE THE PROPERTIES of our foods and medicines. Our tongue is one of our influential teachers when we begin to work with different flavors. Taste—*rasa*, as it's known in Ayurveda—is considered to be the essence of life. We all intuitively know each taste, but we might not have considered what those tastes do. Besides the smell of food, taste is our body's first signal for the digestive system, and smelling and tasting are closely connected. That's why our mouths begin to water when we smell a deliciously aromatic dish. Taste buds tell our digestive system what to prepare for by using enzymes to communicate. Each flavor has an enzymatic quality, which cues our digestive system to respond accordingly.

We can use taste to balance our digestive system as well. For instance, rich flavor in European cuisines often comes from butter and fat. To help offset or balance that heaviness, a raw, bitter salad will often follow the meal, signaling the body to produce more bile to help break down the fat and support digestion. In Indian cultures they often enjoy something sweet before the meal to support the moist quality of the digestive mucosa. Most, if not all, traditional cultures understand how the tastes affect the body.

Recognizing the subtleties of the six tastes will come with practice. Having more awareness or curiosity about the flavors you experience while eating will help you notice more quickly how you feel before, during, and after a meal. This simple practice connects you to your food and the way your body responds to it in a deeper way. If you're experiencing digestive issues of any kind, keeping a food journal (a small notebook that you carry in your bag or even something you keep on your phone) can help you see patterns in your eating habits that may contribute to your issues. This can be especially helpful when working with a practitioner, providing them invaluable clues to where the issues are stemming from.

As you'll see, each taste is created by the elements. Knowing which elements inform the tastes gives you a guide to balancing your own constitution with the flavors that have the opposite effect. So, if you're a person who runs hot physically and digestively, having foods with flavors that are cooling and bitter will benefit you; having foods that are spicy or acidic will aggravate those feelings of heat, and you'll quickly notice that your fire (and possibly your discomfort) has increased after ingesting those foods.

Let's look at each taste and their corresponding elements. While you're reading, notice which flavors call to you the most. Which flavors do you lean on during times of stress? This will give you a clue about the elements that are calling for balance during different times of the year, in different environments, or in different emotional situations.

THE SIX TASTES AND FIVE ELEMENTS

SWEET	=	EARTH + WATER
SOUR	=	EARTH + FIRE
SALTY	=	WATER + FIRE
ASTRINGENT	=	AIR + EARTH
BITTER	=	ETHER + AIR
PUNGENT	=	AIR + FIRE

SWEET: EARTH AND WATER

Sweet, known as *madhura* in Ayurveda, is the most common flavor. It's found in natural sugars and starches such as grains, sweet vegetables and fruits, and herbs such as licorice, marshmallow root, and milky oats. The sweet taste is building, meaning it strengthens body tissue, soothes mucous membranes, and alleviates burning sensations. Sweet foods increase the quality of kapha in the body and promote calmness, contentment, and harmony in the mind. Sweet tastes help vata and pitta constitutions because both doshas need some of the grounding, building, and soothing qualities of kapha.

SOUR: EARTH AND FIRE

Sour flavors are most noticeable in fermented foods and acidic fruits. Some examples are yogurt, miso, pickles, buttermilk, and some sour fruits such as lemons and sour grapes. Herbs such as rose petals, rose hips, and hawthorn berries all have a sour quality. Sour, known as *amla* in Ayurveda, relieves thirst, nourishes, dispels gas, and increases bodily tissues. Sour is good for vata as it will warm, moisten, and ground. Sour can be good for kapha, as it helps break down and liquefy mucus in the digestive system. But too much fermented dairy (a sour taste) can be problematic for kaphas, as dairy is mucus building. Pittas should be wary of too much sour, as it can aggravate the hot quality.

SALTY: WATER ⬠ AND FIRE ⬠

When we talk about the benefits of the salty flavor, we mean foods that are naturally salty, not those flavored with table salt. This flavor, known as *lavana* in Ayurveda, is found in ocean and river salts, seaweed, celery, and herbs such as schisandra berry. Salty foods add moisture and warmth to the body, thus increasing dampness and heat. In small amounts, the salty taste aids digestion, sedates or calms, and softens the body tissues. The vata person, who tends to be cold and dry, will find salty flavors balancing. Pittas and kaphas must stay away from excess salt, especially table salt, because it will aggravate the water and fire qualities within them.

ASTRINGENT: AIR ⬠ AND EARTH ⬠

Astringent can be difficult to experience at first. It's found in foods such as cranberries, apples, and pomegranates and in herbs such as rose petals, witch hazel, and raspberry leaves. Known as *kashaya* in Ayurveda, this taste is drying, stops excess discharges such as sweating and diarrhea, promotes tissue healing, and tones the tissues of the body. It's good for kaphas because it will help dry up excess moisture in the body. It's also good for pittas because it will calm excess heat and reduce moisture and oil.

BITTER: ETHER ⬠ AND AIR ⬠

Once a forgotten flavor, bitter is now making a comeback on menus and in cocktails. It's often found in herbs such as dandelion root and yarrow and foods such as lettuce and swiss chard. It's cooling, drying, and detoxifying, and it contracts bodily tissues, creating lightness both in the body and mind. This taste, known as *tikta* in Ayurveda, will help kapha constitutions because it will lighten and dry up the excess water in their tissues. It's also good for pittas, as it's cooling and will reduce inflammation such as fevers or acidic digestive issues. It's especially good for supporting an aggravated or overheated liver. If you tend to run cold or dry, you will benefit from minimizing your bitter intake, especially in the cold seasons.

PUNGENT: AIR ⬠ AND FIRE ⬠

Pungent flavors are commonly found in warming herbs and spices and vegetables such as mustard greens, radishes, and onions. This flavor, known as *katu* in Ayurveda, is heating, drying, and stimulating, and it increases metabolism, counteracts cold sensations, and aids in digestion. It can be found in some cooling herbs, such as chamomile and lemon balm, as a secondary flavor, meaning that while cooling, they're still stimulating and cleansing. Kaphas can help balance their wet and cold qualities by using generous amounts of pungent spices in their diets. Vatas should use pungent flavors as they're warming but in moderation, as spices such as cayenne or black pepper can be drying. If you tend to run cold and dry, enjoying pungent flavors in liquid, warm, and oily foods such as soups or stews will help reduce the drying effect of this flavor. For pittas who already run hot, spicy and pungent plants, such as ginger and cayenne, should be avoided or consumed in moderation and in relationship to the season.

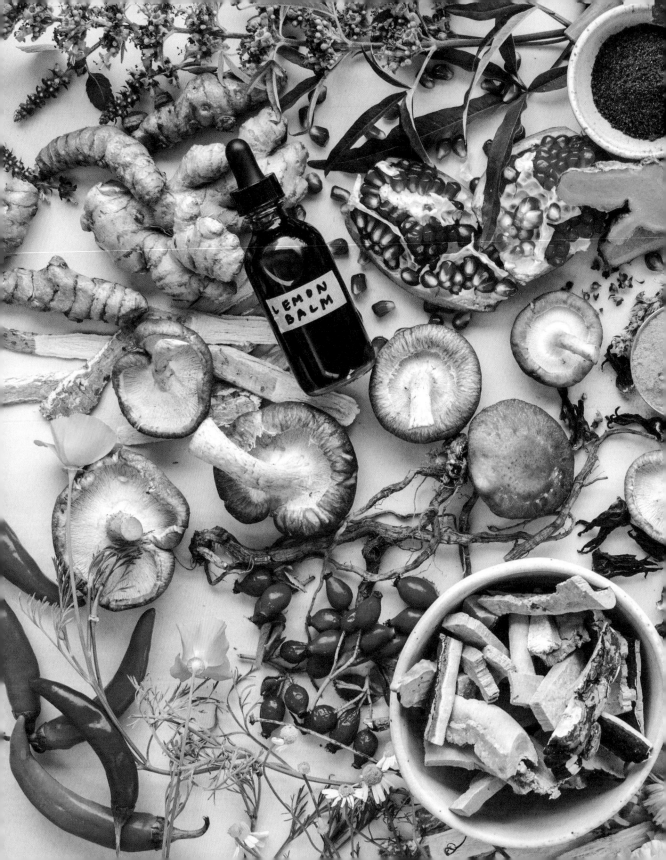

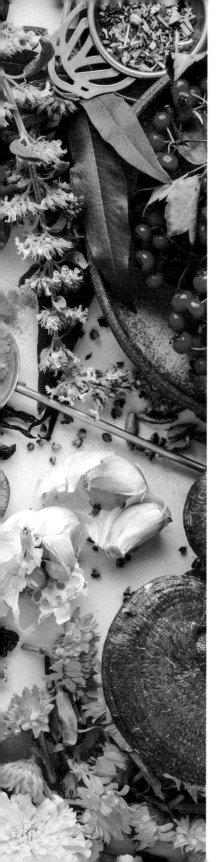

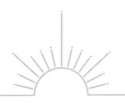

Herbal Actions: How Plants Work on the Body

HERBS OFTEN HAVE HUNDREDS OF CHEMICAL constituents, discovered and identified by modern-day science, and a multitude of herbal actions. Herbal actions are ways of explaining what effects herbs have on the body. Some of these actions are directly related to certain constituents or tastes, such as bitters and their ability to support the gut; other herbal actions work due to a few identifiable constituents and parts still unknown. Science has yet to explain all the mysteries and magic of plant medicines.

While more and more research is being done on plants, most of what we know comes from thousands of years of experiential learning, treatment, and documentation from our ancestors. Isolating plants down to specific chemicals in order to better understand their benefits is new, and herbal research is relatively underfunded (in comparison to Big Pharma), so we're all still learning. And many herbalists believe it's generally less effective to isolate plants down to one single constituent to sell on the marketplace, such as turmeric powder versus curcumin supplements, as it's believed that the plant itself creates more synergy and is more effective when we experience all its components together.

In our herbal glossary you'll find out more about what herbs do, their energetics, how we use them, and the amount suggested for a medicinal dose. You can find the most up-to-date information on dose and safety by researching herbal monographs. We look to publications by the American Botanical Council (ABC) and federal regulating bodies such as Health Canada. Most of the plants we use in our book are rejuvenative tonics and adaptogens, so taking them here and there won't be an issue. But if you want to make significant adjustments, you may wish to buy a scale to measure your herbs and see a practitioner to make sure you're using the right herbs at the best dose.

We've also listed the Latin names as, region to region, many plants share similar common names but are in fact different plants altogether, such as yerba buena in the Americas, which translates to "good herb" and is often a different species with different medicinal effects. If you see "spp." after the first Latin (genus) name, it means we're referring to all plants within that genus. The plant parts are also important to note because many plants have different actions depending on whether you use the root, bark, leaves, flowers, seeds, or berries. As you become a spokesperson for the plants in your community, these nuances will become important.

We have a handy herbal resource guide in the back (page 250) that will show you where we suggest purchasing herbs. It's ideal to grow your own, from a quality and sustainability perspective, but supporting your local herb shops and farmers is another wonderful option. Buying from national (and reputable) herbal companies can also make things easier and more affordable. Please note that in our recipes we indicate what size or cut of herbs and spices to buy, noted by words like ground, powdered, dried, seeds, chips, cut and sifted, and so on.

Safety should always be considered. Herbs are medicine, and they're capable of interacting with pharmaceuticals. In fact, herbs can make medicines more or less effective, and some can even reduce medicines' negative side effects! If you're on any medications or about to undergo surgery, it's important to do your research and communicate with a practitioner about the herbs you're taking.

Above all, remember that plants have unique personalities and energies, just like you. It's important to get to know them and start off slow. It's better to develop a relationship with just a few herbs versus starting off using a ton of medicines at once and becoming confused about what's working. What follows is by no means an exhaustive list but merely the plants we commonly use to keep us feeling well and vibrant. We encourage you to learn more about herbs and connect with an herbalist for more support—see our resources section (page 249) for more information.

ADAPTOGENS

These plants and fungi work to restore overall function and harmony in the body. As they're building and ultimately energizing in nature, they're often warming. Adaptogens work to strengthen and regulate body systems by increasing the body's ability to resist emotional, physical, biological, and environmental stressors. Most adaptogens are believed to work hand in hand with the central nervous system. It usually takes at least a few months of use to feel major changes from the use of adaptogens, especially if the body was initially depleted. It's very important to take adaptogens that fit your dosha or they will not be entirely effective. In the past, many practitioners saw adaptogens as merely normalizing in nature, but we now know some are more like tonics. If you have a major imbalance or illness, it's important to first see a practitioner before tonifying with herbs.

Ashwagandha, astragalus, eleuthero, goji, licorice, maca, reishi, rhodiola, schisandra, shatavari, tulsi

ALTERATIVES

These herbs usually work to restore health by supporting our systems of elimination by way of the kidneys, liver, lungs, and skin. This is usually not a primary action of the herb, but it plays a supportive role in promoting vitality through helping the body move waste out properly. Alterative plants are cleansing, which often makes them cooling energetically. They promote lymphatic flow and reduce inflammation, which can be very helpful to the fiery pittas.

Burdock, cleavers, echinacea, nettle, red clover, turmeric

ANTIMICROBIALS

These herbs inhibit the growth or destroy pathogens such as bacteria, fungi, and viruses. Some of these are culinary herbs but can be used for acute infections such as colds and flus. It can be helpful to use more of these herbs in food or remedies during times when sickness is going around or during the colder months when the body is more susceptible to illness.

Garlic, rosemary, sage, thyme

ANTISPASMODICS

Antispasmodic herbs relieve spasms of voluntary and involuntary muscles. They're often used for reducing the discomfort caused by gas, bloating, cramping, and headaches. Many culinary spices are naturally antispasmodic, which is part of the reason they're so commonly used in foods. Some antispasmodic herbs also fall into the categories of nervines and carminatives, as they help reduce both physical and physiological tension.

Chamomile, ginger, kava kava, passionflower, valerian

ASTRINGENTS

Astringents are correlated with the presence of tannins, which work to tone and tighten tissue, much like the pucker you get when you drink black tea. Astringents are generally used topically (such as witch hazel) for toning the skin, but they can also be used internally to tone and strengthen internal tissues. The astringent taste and herbal action are especially helpful to pittas and kaphas, as the wet qualities benefit from toning and drying qualities.

Blackberry leaf, red raspberry leaf, sage, tea leaf

BITTERS

While bitter is a taste, it's also considered an herbal action. Bitters stimulate the digestive system by activating the liver and gastric juices, so you can better break down and absorb food for nourishment. Bitter flavors can also help you feel full faster, which, in turn, makes you less likely to overeat. They also help normalize blood sugar and help with occasional gas, heartburn, and nausea. It's the forgotten taste that is key to health digestion. Because bitters stimulate and support our processes of elimination, they're great for the liver and skin and for cleansing excess of the wet quality from the body—something that often plagues pittas and kaphas.

Burdock, chamomile, chicory, dandelion, yarrow

CARMINATIVES
Often rich in volatile oils (intense smells), these plants work to promote a healthy digestive system by soothing the digestive tissues and offering relief from cramps, spasms, indigestion, bloating, gas, or nervous stomachs. Depending on the energy of the digestive upset, carminatives can be helpful to all doshas.

Anise, cardamom, chamomile, fennel, peppermint

DEMULCENTS
Plants that are demulcents are high in mucilage, which helps protect and soothe tissues. When used topically, they're called emollients. Internally, these plants protect and heal the lining of our soft tissue mucosa. Because they're often slimy and full of soluble fiber, they can help the digestive system bulk and form soft stool. These actions aid in the promotion of healthy digestive system flow or any ongoing digestive system issues and are great for dry constitutions such as vata. These plants can also be very soothing for folks who have a sore throat.

Calendula, licorice, marshmallow root, mullein, slippery elm

DIAPHORETICS
Nowadays we often avoid a good sweat, but there are traditional remedies that induce sweating to remove toxins. Diaphoretic plants help the body perspire, increasing elimination through the skin. This can be helpful during the early stages of a cold, because perspiration cools the body. Diaphoretics' warming qualities are great for promoting circulation, which helps break up stagnation and mucous that commonly ail kaphas, who often suffer from damp in excess.

Ginger, elderflower, sage, yarrow

EXPECTORANTS
Expectorant plants help the body discharge phlegm and mucus. These herbs can be helpful for stuffy noses and mucus-filled sinuses, which often ail kaphas, who tend to have excess fluid in the body.

Elecampane, eucalyptus, garlic, mullein

NERVINES
These herbs, either tonics or stimulating herbs, work on the nervous system to relax the body and provide relief from stress. Since most modern-day disease is

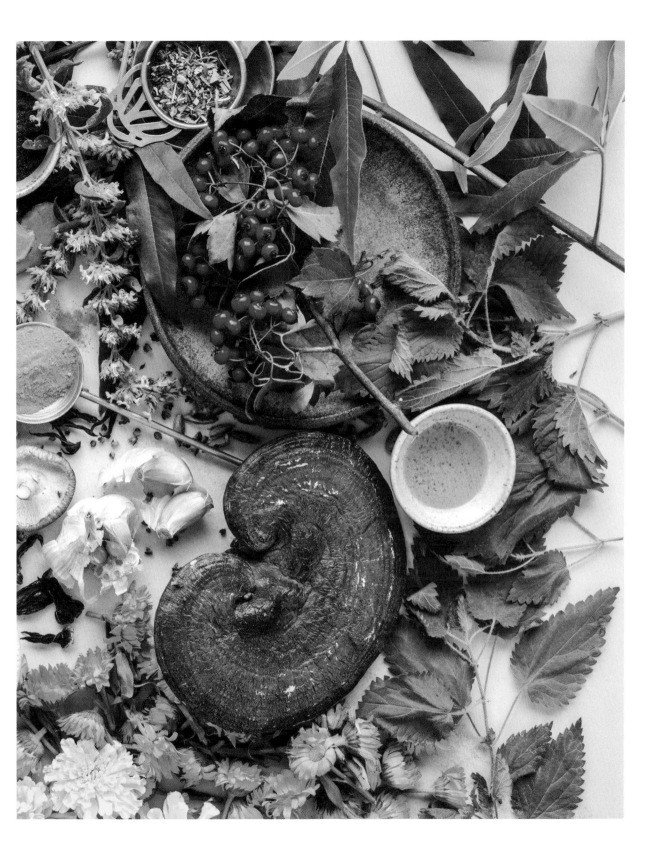

caused by stress, we highly recommend finding a plant ally from this category that you can call on regularly. Once stress is soothed, healing in other parts of the body becomes easier. Since we live in such a stressful world, we believe just about everyone, of any dosha, should be regularly using nervines.

Chamomile, lavender, lemon balm, milky oats, rosemary, skullcap

STIMULANTS

Stimulating herbs are often warming in nature, so they increase internal heat, promoting strong metabolism and circulation through the body. These herbs are great for cold and flu season, stagnation in the body, and cramping. They can also be great to add to food for those who naturally run cold, such as vatas and kaphas.

Cayenne, cinnamon, ginger, thyme

TONICS

Tonic plants enhance the function and overall vitality of body systems by strengthening them. They may increase energy, but unlike stimulants (such as coffee), they promote vigor without negative side effects. This energy is generally restored through using tonics over time and building the health of the body system. Unlike adaptogens, they generally are body-system specific, meaning they provide a focused effort versus an overall normalizing effect.

There are cardiac tonics (hawthorn berries), digestive system tonics (dandelion leaf and root), nervous system tonics (skullcap), and reproductive system tonics (raspberry leaf, for those with ovaries)—just to name a few. There are specific herbal tonics that can be used to support every system in the body.

Please note that some adaptogens can be considered tonics, as they alleviate weakness and promote the vitality of specific systems, but not all tonics are considered adaptogens. Adaptogens have broader effects and are less specific to one particular body system.

Dandelion, hawthorn, milky oat, nettle, raspberry, skullcap

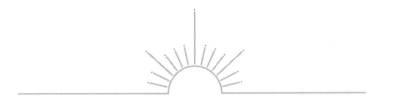

In the Kitchen

Stocking Your Kitchen Apothecary

All herbs and spices, even those often seen only as tools for flavor, are actually medicinal. Our ancestors used these plants to not only create delicious food but also support the body throughout the seasons. Looking to your spice rack for everyday support is a building block of creating a healing kitchen. You will notice that many of the dried herbs and spices we use tend to be warming and stimulating to the digestive system, which will be helpful for those who have less digestive fire or who are seeking warmth during the cooler months of the year. Here are some of our favorites, and likely yours too, along with ways to use them every day.

BLACK PEPPER (*Piper nigrum*) This common everyday seasoning is a powerful digestive aid that helps warm the digestive system to break down and assimilate food properly. It can be quite warming, so use sparingly if you tend to run hot. Black pepper mixed with honey makes a wonderful expectorant, which helps move out and dry up excess mucus.

Try it in medicinal honey, or sprinkled on food for its warming properties.

CARDAMOM (*Elettaria cardamomum*) This slightly warming and stimulating spice can help move excess mucus. It's widely known for its digestive supporting actions and its help with heartburn, bloating, and gas. You can also chew on cardamom seeds to get a little natural breath freshener.

Try it in our Adaptogenic Luna Chai (page 188), Kava Kava White Russian (page 155), Kosmic Kitchen Sink Cookies with Goji, Maca, and Dark Chocolate (page 208), Cardamom Basmati Rice (page 232), tea, coffee, warm milk, and rice.

CAYENNE (*Capsicum annuum*) A warming and stimulating pepper, cayenne is great for overall circulation and is a diaphoretic. It's activating and helps to balance when there is an excess of cold or wet qualities.

Try it in our Fire Cider Elixir (page 222), Spicy Mushroom Hot Cacao (page 225), and broths.

CINNAMON (*Cinnamomum spp.*) This warming and harmonizing spice is also great for circulation. It promotes cardiovascular health and is often used to promote healthy blood sugar levels.

Try it on our sweet Overnight Oats (page 127), in Ashwagandha Turmeric Golden Milk Elixir (page 187), Everyday Fall Brew (page 186), or with roasted root vegetables, squash, and porridge.

CORIANDER (*Coriandrum sativum*) A warming, bitter, and astringent spice that comes from the cilantro plant when it goes to seed. As a carminative, it helps to soothe digestive upset such as bloating, gas, and indigestion. This spice is great to chew on, infuse into soups and curries, or create a tea to support digestion.

Try it in our Kosmic Kurry Spice Blend (page 99).

CUMIN (*Cuminum cyminum*) Slightly warming, bitter, and pungent, this seed is an enzymatic carminative that helps the body break down and better absorb nutrients. It's also high in vitamin C and has antifungal properties. As an antispasmodic, it's great for indigestion and cramping.

Try it in our Kosmic Kurry Spice Blend (page 99), Magical Mushroom Mole (page 197), or to season beans.

FENNEL (*Foeniculum vulgare*) A sweet and cooling seed, fennel is great for stomachaches, cramping, and spasms in the digestive system. It can be chewed after meals or included in curries and soups for extra digestive support.

Try it in our Minty Holiday Tea (page 221), Kitchari Blend (page 100), in curry, or just toasted and chewed for a postmeal digestive aid.

GARLIC (*Allium sativum*) Sour and heating, garlic is said to work on all tissues. It's a stimulant, antimicrobial, and expectorant, making it great for colds and coughs. It helps to move mucus out of the body.

Try it in our Fire Cider Elixir (page 222) or in Ginger–Garlic Braised Dandelion Greens (page 129).

GINGER (*Zingiber officinale*) A pungent and heating rhizome, ginger is great for circulation and warming and activating any food or formula. It works wonders on digestive system upsets and helps relieve gas and bloating after a large meal. It's also an antispasmodic, making it great for menstrual cramps. As a diaphoretic, it helps the body sweat out mild fevers.

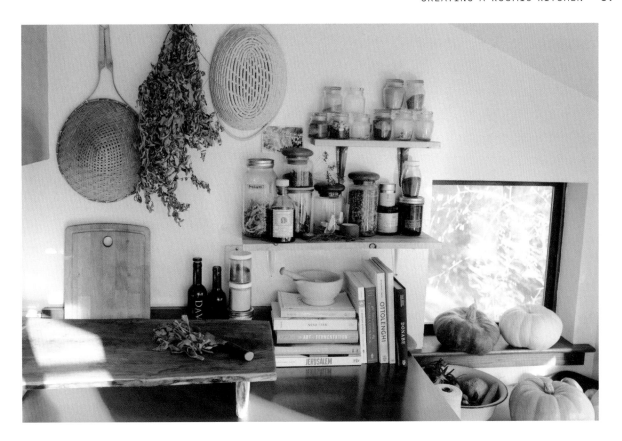

Use it in our Adaptogenic Luna Chai (page 188) or Fire Cider Elixir (page 222), Ginger Persimmon Oat Bars (page 238), Tom Kha Gai with Rice Noodles with Lemon Balm (page 191), as an addition to our Ashwagandha Turmeric Golden Milk Elixir (page 187), and in everyday broths.

ROSEMARY (*Rosmarinus officinalis*) This bitter, pungent, and warming Mediterranean herb is also an antimicrobial that's great for colds and flus and is famously known for its memory-enhancing properties. We also love using it to support the nervous system, especially in the cold times of year accompanied by stress.

Use it in teas, in Herbal Steams (page 146), teas, with roasted vegetables, or in a dressing.

SAGE (*Salvia officinalis*) Culinary sage is astringent, bitter, pungent, and warming. It's often a helpful herb for menopause. In Western herbalism it's commonly used in tea with honey for congestion, sore throats, colds, and flus.

Use it in Herbal Honey (page 108), in teas, as a throat gargle, in stews, or sautéed with mushrooms.

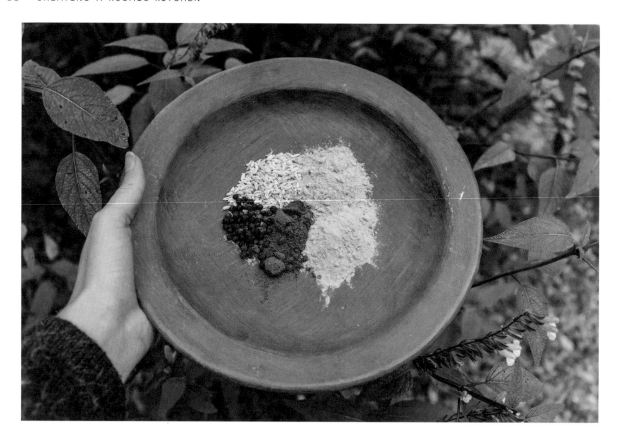

THYME (*Thymus vulgaris*) Heating and pungent, thyme is commonly used in traditional European tea blends, syrups, and other formulas to help with colds and flus in the depths of winter. It's an antibacterial and has been used throughout history to ward off sickness.

Try using it in Herbal Steams (page 146), Everyday Herbal Bone Broth (page 112), marinades, winter salads, herbal syrups, and teas.

TURMERIC (*Curcuma longa*) This is a bitter, pungent, and heating herb that does more than most and (in our opinion) is worth all the hype. It supports the digestive system by helping the body break down and absorb food more easily. It supports the circulatory and immune systems, and it's great for inflammation pain. It can also be used as an alterative to help our lymphatic system health and give the skin an extra glow.

Try it in our Turmeric Tahini Dressing (page 105), Kosmic Kurry Spice Blend (page 99), Ashwagandha Turmeric Golden Milk Elixir (page 187), Turmeric Spice Honey (page 109), or in Turmeric Congee (page 226).

Healing Plants for the Kosmic Pantry

This book focuses on herbs that can be easily found in the grocery store, farmers market, or online. We've also selected herbs that we've developed relationships with over the years, those that have provided healing and comfort for us in times of need. Because our herbal practice revolves around the kitchen, most of the herbs we use can weave seamlessly into dishes once you get to know their actions, energetic profiles, and flavors.

We encourage you to get to know your local ecosystems so that you can develop a relationship with your local plants and create a bioregional practice—maybe you can even grow your own! This book is meant to provide an elemental lens to your practice so you can ultimately be creative with whatever you have handy.

Some of these plants have more medicinal parts than we've listed. We've chosen to highlight how we most frequently use the plants to keep things clear and easy. So, don't be surprised if you find something new and interesting about these plants elsewhere; there could be a whole book on the powers of these incredible medicines. There are an untold number of herbal remedies; we're sharing the remedies we feel are most relevant for everyday kitchen herbalism. This way, you can easily understand which plants work well for which common ailments, and you can discover the abilities of many plants you may already use.

We've also referenced professional monographs for proper dosage, which is why the measurements are mostly in grams. Dosages are important to consider in order to get enough of the herbs to have an effect on the body. Sometimes when starting to use herbal medicine, folks think these remedies are similar to the allopathic model of taking one pill a day to feel the effects. Plant medicine is quite different in that regard; you must form a relationship with these medicines, working with them over time. This book mostly focuses on rejuvenative herbs that are (more or less) traditionally used in foods to promote vitality and prevent illness. If

Dried rosehips

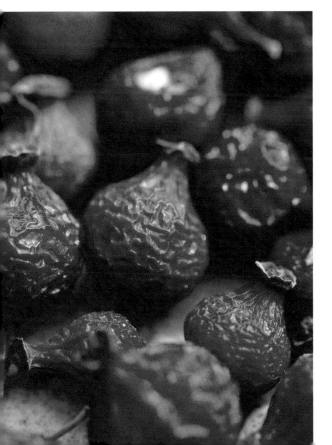

you're working with an herb for a specific effect or an ongoing issue, then please keep in mind the layer of dosage and work with a practitioner.

If it took months or even years to get out of balance, it will take time for these plant medicines to work with your body. A typical rule of thumb is to work with an herb or herbal formula for three months to give your body time to respond. Use the dosages and recipes we provide as a guide to the amount you need to feel an effect over time, adding them to foods and beverages daily. We've given suggestions on how to use the herbs based on their flavor and energetics, and there's more on that in the recipe sections in part 3. As you begin to use herbs at home, it may be helpful to purchase a kitchen scale and start with a small amount so you know exactly how much herb you're getting. However, most of our recipes include simple teaspoon and tablespoon measurements for ease of use; if we use other forms of measurement like quart and pint jars, it's to allude to the fact that the recipe will also be filled and used for storage of your kitchen medicine.

ASHWAGANDHA (Withania somnifera)

ENERGETICS: Warming and slightly drying, bitter, sweet

PARTS USED: Root

BENEFITS: As a member of the Solanaceae (or nightshade) family, along with peppers and tomatoes, ashwagandha is warming. These warming properties stimulate metabolism and digestion, clear excess mucus, and improve circulation. Ashwagandha is also an adaptogen in Western herbalism, or a rasayana (rejuvenative tonic) in Ayurveda. This powerful root promotes restful sleep, reduces anxiety and depression, revitalizes low libido, and soothes arthritic inflammation. The sweet and building properties are nutritive and help restore proper hormone function and nourish the nervous system. Ashwagandha can be taken in a warm milky tea with cardamom or cinnamon before bed to promote sleep. It's one of the few adaptogens that can have an immediate calming effect, especially when mixed with grounding foods such as milk, dairy or otherwise. A couple of our favorite ways to enjoy the benefits of this plant are in our Herbal Power Bites (page 114) and Ashwagandha Turmeric Golden Milk Elixir (page 187).

DOSAGE: 2 to 6 grams of dried powdered root throughout the day. Mix the powdered root in warm beverages, dips, or mixed seed butter and honey for a sweet snack.

SAFETY: Avoid if pregnant or trying to get pregnant.

ASTRAGALUS (Astragalus membranaceus)

ENERGETICS: Warming and moistening, sweet

PARTS USED: Root

BENEFITS: Considered a primary herb in Chinese medicine, astragalus is an adaptogen, or chi tonic, used for those under immunological stress or who have a weakened immune system. Its warming and sweet properties stimulate metabolism

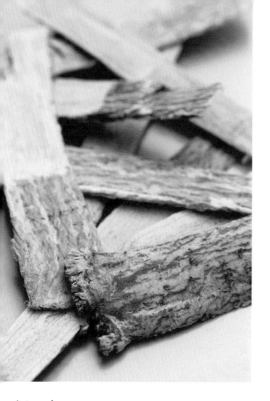

Astragalus

and digestion. Astragalus has also been heavily researched in the field of oncology and often plays a supportive role in cancer treatment programs. We like to use a few slices of dried root when cooking our Turmeric Congee (page 226) or making Everyday Herbal Bone Broth (page 112).

SAFETY: If you're taking immunosuppressive drugs, have an autoimmune disease, or are undergoing cancer treatment, it's best to consult with a practitioner before use.

DOSAGE: 2.25 to 5 grams throughout the day. Mix the powdered root in warm beverages, dips, seed-butter snacks, or 3 to 4 dried slices in a batch of broth.

BURDOCK (*Arctium lappa*)

ENERGETICS: Cooling and moistening, bitter, sweet

PARTS USED: Root

BENEFITS: Heat-clearing burdock is known to reduce swelling and inflammation both internally and externally. As an alterative and demulcent in Western herbalism, it's often used to clear and soothe skin conditions such as acne, eczema, psoriasis, and boils. Overall, it's wonderful for the lymphatic system and dry skin conditions. Also known as *gobo* in Japanese, burdock is enjoyed in many Asian cuisines as pickles and in sushi and stir-fry. Look for the fresh root in most Asian specialty markets. We use burdock in our Herbal Vinegars (page 104) and Miso Immune Soup with Astragalus, Burdock, and Shiitake (page 229).

DOSAGE: 1.2 to 18 grams of dried root throughout the day. It goes great in tea, infused in vinegar, or sliced thin and sautéed for a snack.

CALENDULA (*Calendula officinalis*)

ENERGETICS: Warming and drying, slightly bitter, salty, sweet

PARTS USED: Flower

BENEFITS: Calendula, also called pot marigold, creates resinous yellow and orange flowers that hold an incredible vulnerary (wound healing) power that's soothing to internal and external tissues. It works to calm inflamed mucous membranes, making it a great tea for those dealing with hot, dry, and depleted digestive systems with compromised gut tissues. It's often infused into oils and creams for topical use, to support the healing of skin issues, minor wounds and burns, and bruising. It yields a beautiful golden hue, which gives the skin a radiant glow. It's also great for the lymphatic system and can be a wonderful addition to an internal formula for skin. We love using fresh calendula as an edible flower garnish or infusing the dried flowers in soups and teas to bring radiance into the depths of winter. Try it in our Everyday Spring Brew (page 122), Flower Power Honey (page 140), or Herbal Steams (page 146).

DOSAGE: 0.18 to 12 grams of dried flower throughout the day. Calendula is lovely enjoyed as a tea or infused in honey.

CHAMOMILE (*Matricaria chamomilla*)

ENERGETICS: Slightly cooling, pungent, bitter

PARTS USED: Flower

BENEFITS: As a nervine and antispasmodic, chamomile is used to soothe emotional and muscle tension and promote a sense of calm. It's also a carminative that's especially helpful for stress manifesting in the gut in the form of excess gas, cramping, IBS, and ulcers. It's also calming to heat-related emotional and physical issues, such as anger, frustration, and eczema. We love using it in baths, teas, and as an herbal garnish. Try it in our Summer Berry Crumble with Chamomile and Lavender Coconut Cream (page 174) or Lavender, Chamomile, and Skullcap Cooler (page 153).

DOSAGE: 1.5 to 24 grams of dried flower throughout the day. Enjoy as a relaxing tea during the day or make a strong cup to promote restful sleep before bed.

CHASTE TREE (*Vitex agnus-castus*)

ENERGETICS: Warming and drying, bitter

PARTS USED: Berry

BENEFITS: Vitex, or chaste berry, is a hormonal normalizer that works to harmonize the pituitary gland, more specifically in regard to progesterone levels. As both a hormone regulator and uterine tonic, this herb often comes in handy to those experiencing cycle irregularity or loss of menses due to discontinuing oral contraceptives. It's also beneficial for general hormone-related issues such as menstrual cramping, PMS, and menopausal symptoms. Try it in our Adaptogenic Luna Chai (page 188).

SAFETY: Please avoid if you're on birth control or hormone-related drugs, and consult your practitioner before using if you have a hormone-related disorder. When taking dopamine-related medications, it's also best to avoid; or speak with a professional.

DOSAGE: 0.4 to 0.8 grams throughout the day. We love infusing chaste berries in a rich, rooty tea blend with lots of warming spices.

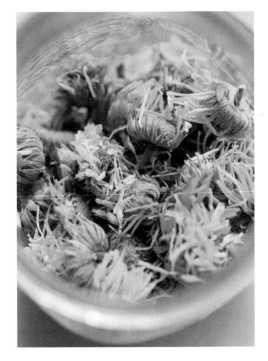

Calendula

DANDELION (Taraxacum officinale)

ENERGETICS: Cooling and drying, bitter

PARTS USED: Root, leaf, and flower

BENEFITS: Dandelion is known as an incredible tonic, and every part of it is considered medicinal. The greens are rich in vitamins A, C, and K, iron, calcium, potassium, and more. They're also a prebiotic, made up of a unique type of fiber that only exists in certain plants. The leaves contain powerful diuretic properties, which help the kidneys maintain balance through supporting elimination of excess fluids. The roots are known as a liver tonic and support digestion by stimulating the liver and digestive enzymes. This helps the body break down foods to better assimilate what we need and eliminate what we don't. By supporting the systems of elimination and detoxification, dandelion is also helpful to the skin. Try it in our Everyday Fall Brew (page 186) or in our Roasted Dandelion Chai Concentrate (page 125).

DOSAGE: 12 to 30 grams of dried leaf, 6 to 24 grams of dried root. We use the dried roots for their rich flavor as a base for "liver teas" or we infuse fresh roots to make an herbal vinegar.

ELDERBERRY (Sambucus nigra)

ENERGETICS: Cooling and moistening, bitter

PARTS USED: Berry and flower

BENEFITS: The flower and berry of the elder tree are both known as diaphoretics in Western herbalism, meaning that they help the body break a sweat, which can be useful in early stages of a cold, flu, or illness. While seemingly counterintuitive, in traditional medicine this perspiration helps cool the body and catalyze healing. The flower is also an antispasmodic, making it great for ongoing coughs. Try it in our Everyday Winter Berry Brew (page 220).

DOSAGE: 1.5 to 15 grams of dried flowers throughout the day, 1.3 to 18 grams of dried berries throughout the day. The berries make a delicious tea, or infuse the berries into a syrup.

ELEUTHERO (Eleutherococcus senticosus)

ENERGETICS: Warming, slightly bitter, pungent

PARTS USED: Root

BENEFITS: As an adaptogen, eleuthero, or Siberian ginseng, works to return balance to the entire body. Over time, the user is able to better respond to stress both internally and externally. Because of its warming nature, it's ideal for those who are running on overdrive and running cold. This could offer support to those with ongoing fear, trauma, anxiety, and depression. As with many adaptogens, eleuthero is often used for those suffering from chronic illness who have a suppressed immune and weakened nervous system, under a professional's care. Try it in our Herbal Power Bites (page 114) or Turmeric Spice Honey (page 109).

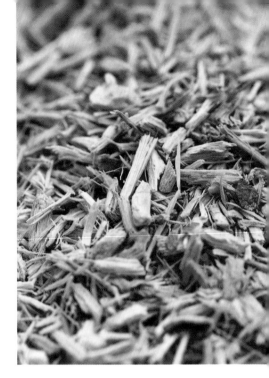

Eleuthero

DOSAGE: 2 to 3 grams of powdered herb throughout the day. Mix the powdered root with hot water and honey for a quick tea or mix with seed butter and honey for a quick sweet treat.

HAWTHORN (*Crataegus spp.*)

ENERGETICS: Slightly warming, sour, sweet

PARTS USED: Berry and leaves

BENEFITS: Hawthorn is traditionally a symbol of love, and in more recent times it has been clinically proven to support the heart and cardiovascular system as a cardiotonic. The berries work to improve overall circulation, strengthen the heart, and normalize the heartbeat. Try it in our Ginger Persimmon Oat Bars (page 238) or Spiced Mulled Wine with Hawthorn Berries (page 190).

SAFETY: This herb can enhance the effects of cardiovascular drugs, so it's best to speak with a practitioner before use if you have any heart health concerns.

DOSAGE: 0.6 to 3.5 grams of dried berry throughout the day. The berries are delicious in tea blends or infused into a syrup.

HIBISCUS (*Hibiscus sabdariffa*)

ENERGETICS: Cooling, sour, slightly sweet

PARTS USED: Calyx

BENEFITS: Hibiscus, or roselle, has been used traditionally in North Africa, Southeast Asia, and more recently in the Caribbean and Central America as both a refreshing beverage and cardiotonic. It primarily promotes healthy circulation and normalizes blood pressure when used over time. Try it in our Fire Cider Elixir (page 222) or Hibiscus Punch with Schisandra Salt Rims (page 156).

DOSAGE: 1.25 to 10 grams throughout the day. In the summer months, we love refreshing hibiscus tea sprinkled with edible flowers.

KAVA KAVA (*Piper methysticum*)

ENERGETICS: Warming and drying, pungent

PARTS USED: Rhizome

BENEFITS: As both a nervine and hypnotic, kava kava primarily works to soothe and calm the nervous system. Traditionally it's used in ceremony in the Fijian islands. These days you can find it in kava bars, teas, and pills to promote relaxation. It's especially helpful for those suffering from ongoing anxiety and/or depression. As an antispasmodic, this rhizome is very helpful for severe cramps and pain. Try it in our Kava Kava White Russian (page 155).

SAFETY: It's one of the strongest herbs for anxiety so it's important to work with a practitioner to determine the proper dose if used over time. It can create a drunken feeling if consumed in large quantities, so please use this herb in moderation and, with continued use, under supervision of a practitioner. Avoid if pregnant or trying to get pregnant.

DOSAGE: 1.7 to 3.4 grams of dried rhizome throughout the day, best used in low doses to start. It makes a delicious tea, especially when paired with warming spices and coconut milk.

LEMON BALM (Melissa officinalis)

ENERGETICS: Cooling, sweet, pungent

PARTS USED: Leaves and flowers

BENEFITS: Most widely used for its ability to soothe and calm the digestive and nervous systems, lemon balm is one of our favorite nervines. Its antibacterial and antiviral properties make it an ally for those suffering from cold sores by helping reduce not only the infection but also the stress that causes flare-ups. It grows prolifically in the spring and summer, and the leaves and flowers are most potent when used fresh. Lemon balm goes great in our Boozy Lemon Balm Cooler (page 143) and Lemon Balm Gazpacho with Za'atar Quinoa and Cucumber Salad (page 165).

DOSAGE: 1.5 to 4.5 grams of dried herb, 1 to 3 times per day. Add fresh leaves to make tea, pesto, syrups, vinegars, and dressings.

SAFETY: Please consult a practitioner if you have hypothyroidism.

LICORICE (Glycyrrhiza glabra, Glycyrrhiza uralensis)

ENERGETICS: Warming and moistening, sweet, slightly bitter

PARTS USED: Root

BENEFITS: This sweet-tasting root supports the endocrine system. It's also an adaptogen with an affinity for supporting the body during burnout or fatigue and as a support for the adrenals to help prevent burnout. Enjoy licorice as a tea in the afternoon to curb cravings for sweets when it's common to feel sluggish. Its demulcent properties are wonderful to soothe sore throats and inflamed tissues of the digestive and respiratory systems. It's well known in Chinese medicine for being a harmonizing herb, helping make formulas more palatable and balanced. Try it in our Everyday Spring Brew (page 122) or add to Fire Cider Elixir (page 222).

DOSAGE: 0.6 to 15 grams per day of dried herb or powder. We like to add the powder to seed-butter snacks, desserts, or in hot water for a quick tea.

SAFETY: Not recommended to use if you have high blood pressure, kidney or cardiovascular disorder, or if you're taking medications that aggravate electrolyte imbalances. Avoid if pregnant or trying to get pregnant. Please consult your health-care practitioner before using if you have any of the conditions mentioned above.

MACA (*Lepidium meyenii*)

ENERGETICS: Warming, sweet, slightly bitter

PARTS USED: Root

BENEFITS: Maca root, endemic to the Andes of Peru and Bolivia, has long been a traditional food source for its high nutritional content of amino acids, vitamins, fiber, and fatty acids. This warming, slightly sweet, and nutty-flavored root is used to promote stamina, fertility, and healthy libido while helping bring balance to the endocrine system. Try it in our Adaptogenic Ginger Maca Miso Dressing (page 106), Date and Nut Apple Pie Bites (page 202), or our Kosmic Kitchen Sink Cookies with Goji, Maca, and Dark Chocolate (page 208).

DOSAGE: 0.06 to 3.5 grams per day of powder. Its malty flavor pairs well in hot beverages, seedbutters, and desserts.

NETTLE (*Urtica diocia*)

ENERGETICS: Cooling and drying, astringent

PARTS USED: Leaves

BENEFITS: One of the most tonifying herbs prized by herbalists, nettle is rich in chlorophyll, vitamins, and minerals such as iron, manganese, zinc, calcium, potassium, and others. It has an affinity for the genitourinary tract and helps to support and strengthen the kidneys, an important source of the body's energy. Used for liver support, nettle helps aid in the symptoms of seasonal allergies when taken as freeze-dried capsules. Try it in our Wild Weeds Pesto (page 102) or in our Nourishing Nettle Soup with White Beans and Shiitakes (page 134).

DOSAGE: 2 to 5 grams, 3 times per day. We love nettle fresh or dried as a simple tea, blended in dressings, in an herbal vinegar, or steamed and eaten like greens.

PASSIONFLOWER (*Passiflora incarnata*)

ENERGETICS: Bitter, cooling, pungent

PARTS USED: Leaves and flowers

BENEFITS: Passionflower vine has striking blooms but its medicine lies in its leaves. One of the most revered nervines, passionflower is often given to soothe restless minds from anxiety and insomnia. It's commonly used for its sedating effects, though not everyone reacts to it this way. Its antispasmodic action makes it an ally for menstrual cramps or spasms in the muscles. Try it in our Everyday Summer Brew (page 152).

DOSAGE: 1 to 2 grams dried aerial parts, 1 to 4 times per day. We enjoy passionflower tea to help quiet the mind before bed or combined with other anxiety-relieving nervines to sip on throughout the day.

PEPPERMINT (*Mentha x piperita*)

ENERGETICS: Pungent, cooling

PARTS USED: Leaves

BENEFITS: Peppermint is one of the most refreshing digestive aids to help relieve gas, bloating, and nausea. Its diaphoretic, or sweating, action can be helpful to use during colds and flus. We often add peppermint in herbal tea formulas to balance the flavor of other less pleasant-tasting plants. Try it in our Minty Holiday Tea (page 221).

DOSAGE: 1 to 4 grams, 3 times a day. Use fresh peppermint sparingly in tea formulas, in pesto, yogurt dips, dressings, and desserts.

SAFETY: Though this herb is known for its digestive soothing properties, it's best to avoid with GERD or heartburn as it can be too relaxing and cause acid to pour back into the esophagus from the stomach, making those symptoms worse.

RED CLOVER (*Trifolium pratense*)

ENERGETICS: Bitter, sweet, cooling, pungent

PARTS USED: Leaves and flowers

BENEFITS: This low-lying herb is a wonderful respiratory tonic that helps soothe coughs and colds. Because of its high mineral content as calcium, nitrogen, and iron, red clover is often found in reproductive formulas as a nutritive, helping support and purify the blood. Its detoxifying blood-purifying properties help clear skin conditions as well as cysts and fibroids from the body. Try it in a Hot Water Herbal Infusion (page 94) along with herbs like nettle and burdock root in springtime.

DOSAGE: 250 milligrams to 1 gram, leaves and flowers, 3 times a day in a tea.

CONTRAINDICATIONS: If taking blood-thinning medication or hormone replacement therapy, consult a practitioner.

REISHI (*Ganoderma lucidum*)

ENERGETICS: Bitter, warming

PARTS USED: Fruiting body

BENEFITS: Once a rare herb only used by Chinese royalty, reishi has been known to nourish the heart, which stores *shen*, a person's emotional balance and mind or consciousness. When our shen is disturbed or out of balance, we can experience anxiety, insomnia, moodiness, and poor memory. It has been used in the folk medicine of China and Japan for over two thousand years and has been documented to use for its support around degenerative conditions and for promoting longevity. We use reishi acutely for allergy season and more long term for its adaptogenic properties known for boosting vitality and nourishing the heart. Try it in our Raw Reishi Mousse Cups (page 177) and Reishi Rose Chocolate Bark (page 241).

DOSAGE: 3 to 15 grams dried extracted powder in desserts, hot chocolate, or as a coffee alternative.

ROSE (Rosa spp.)

ENERGETICS: Bitter, pungent, astringent, sweet, cooling

PARTS USED: Flowers

BENEFITS: This sweet flower is an ally for reducing heat in the body, while its astringent properties help soothe inflamed skin and tissues. Energetically, rose helps open the heart to bring forth a sense of ease and self-love. It also has an affinity for the female reproductive system, helping ease cramps and regulate menstruation. Try it in our Rose Cinnamon Tahini Milk (page 126), Everyday Spring Brew (page 122), or Reishi Rose Chocolate Bark (page 241).

DOSAGE: 250 milligrams to 1 gram dried rose petals. Use in teas and sweets, or in a bath or facial steam.

SCHISANDRA (Schisandra chinensis)

ENERGETICS: Warming and drying

PARTS USED: Berries

BENEFITS: Known as the five-flavor fruit, schisandra berries are sour, sweet, bitter, astringent, and pungent. Schisandra is beneficial for controlling frequent urination and drying up excess fluids, along with having anti-inflammatory properties that are beneficial for soothing asthma and wet coughs. As an adaptogen, it has a dual effect on the nervous system, meaning it has mild stimulating qualities and it helps reduce anxiety and promote calming. Studies have shown the berries to be beneficial in normalizing blood pressure. Try it in our Hibiscus Punch with Schisandra Salt Rims (page 156) or Everyday Winter Berry Brew (page 220).

DOSAGE: 1 to 6 grams a day of powder or dried berries decocted. Enjoy as a tart addition to dressings, teas, or dips.

SAFETY: Schisandra can interact with some prescription drugs, similar to grapefruit juice. Consult your pharmacist or health-care provider if you're taking prescription drugs.

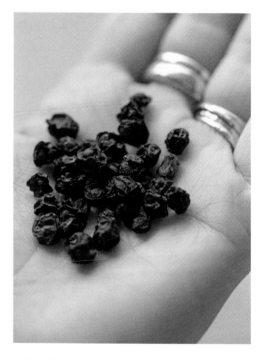

Schisandra

SHATAVARI (Asparagus racemosus)

ENERGETICS: Cooling and moistening, sweet, bitter

PARTS USED: Root

BENEFITS: A prized plant in Ayurveda, its name means "she who has hundreds of husbands." While that sounds like a lot to us, the lore alludes to the root's affinity for the female reproductive system. The moistening and cooling energy of the root is used to promote reproductive health (males included), a healthy libido, hormone balance, and milk production. It also works to boost the immune system and energy

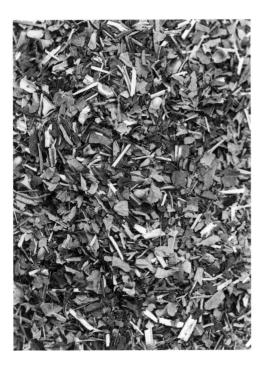

Skullcap

levels and soothe the digestive system. It goes well in ghee, warm milk, or as a tea with a bit of fat. Try it in our Kosmic Kurry Spice Blend (page 99) or Adaptogenic Ghee-Stuffed Dates (page 139).

DOSAGE: 1 to 3 grams daily of the powder in tea or seed-butter bites or mixed with ghee.

SKULLCAP (*Scutellaria lateriflora*)

ENERGETICS: Bitter, cooling

PARTS USED: Leaves and flowers

BENEFITS: A prized nervine that helps strengthen the brain and revitalize the central nervous system, skullcap helps calm the mind and relieve nervous stress. Its antispasmodic properties help relax nervous tension and headaches. It's a wonderful nervine to use throughout the day, as it doesn't tend to make you drowsy, but rather calm and focused. Try it in our Lavender, Chamomile, and Skullcap Cooler (page 153).

DOSAGE: 250 milligrams to 1 gram a day as a tea.

TULSI (*Ocimun tenuiflorum*)

ENERGETICS: Warming and drying, sweet, pungent

PARTS USED: Leaves and flowers

BENEFITS: Tulsi, also known as holy basil, is one of the most delicious-tasting adaptogens. It's highly regarded in Ayurveda for its ability to calm the nervous system and uplift one's spirit. Tulsi flourishes in intense heat (dry or humid) and can easily be grown in a pot outdoors. Herbalist David Winston uses tulsi in his practice to relieve mental fog, stagnant depression, and allergies to mold and animal dander. Modern studies show tulsi to be effective in lowering blood sugar levels, protecting against ionizing radiation, and decreasing stress hormone levels. Try it in our Wild Weeds Pesto (page 102) or Everyday Summer Brew (page 152).

DOSAGE: 4 grams or 1 teaspoon of dried leaves as a tea, throughout the day. We use the fresh leaves alone or in combination with other herbs in pesto, as you would sweet basil.

SAFETY: Avoid if pregnant or trying to get pregnant, as some studies have shown antifertility activity.

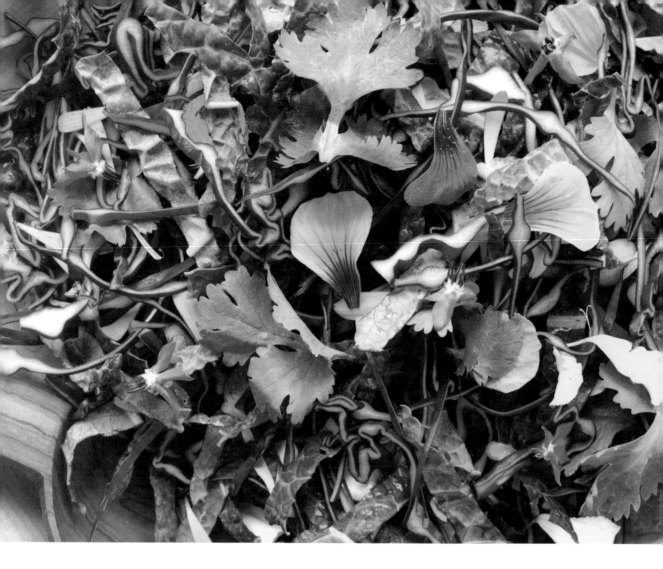

Edible Flowers

Edible flowers are a fun way to introduce people to the magic of plants. Few can resist the draw of flowers adorning a dish. They're food for the eyes and the soul. In the height of summer, our kitchens are scattered with yellow, pink, red, and blue blooms ready to be sprinkled in salads, dips, drinks, and sweets. From snapdragon and sage flowers to fava flowers, mustards, and sunflower petals, summer is bursting with Mother Nature's confetti. While there are many edible flowers, we've listed a few of our favorites that are easy to find or grow. When seeking out flowers you can eat, it's important to make sure you're able to safely identify them before ingesting.

NASTURTIUM FLOWERS AND LEAVES (*Tropaeolum majus*)

Probably the most well-known edible flower, nasturtiums are commonly found growing in many gardens across the world. Different varieties yield plants that tend to climb or seem more vine-like, while others will fill out to look more like a low-growing bush. The flowers can range in hue from deep red to variegated peach and yellow to the more commonly seen bright orange.

FLAVOR: Spicy! A little kick of spicy mustard that's perfect for adding to savory dishes or sweet ones if you're looking for some contrast. We like to separate the petals, so the flavor isn't as intense. The leaves, which share the spicy flavor of the flowers, also make nice additions to salads or can be used for garnish.

ABUTILON FLOWERS (*Abutilon pictum*)

As members of the Malvaceae (mallow) family, these lantern-shaped flowers are on the larger end of the edible flower spectrum. Often seen in hues of orange, red, or yellow, abutilons are a fun addition to sweet and savory dishes.

FLAVOR: Slightly sweet and astringent. Since they can be large, separate the petals when mixing them into a dish. These go really well in citrus salads or as part of a larger decorative addition to cakes and sweets.

BORAGE FLOWERS AND LEAVES (*Borago officinalis*)

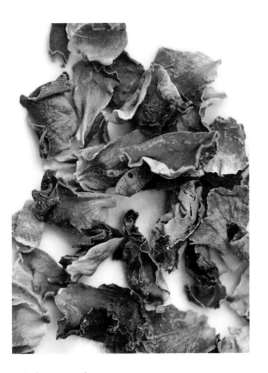

These bluish-purple flowers are friends of the bees. Planted in a garden, they provide brilliant pops of color amidst the hues of green. Medicinally, borage is used for uplifting the spirit and helping reduce anxiety and depression.

FLAVOR: Pleasantly mild and unexpectedly tastes like cucumber! Use the flowers on your favorite dishes or the fresh leaves muddled in water for a cucumber-kissed drink.

CALENDULA FLOWERS (*Calendula officinalis*)

These cheery blooms are found in most herbalists' gardens. On the medicinal side, they're true healers, helping soothe cuts and bruises as well as soft tissues in the digestive tract. While a sprinkle or two isn't a large enough dose to feel the effects, their bright color surely brings joy to any occasion. The flowers range in hues from bright yellow to rusty orange, and they love to be harvested often to encourage even more flowers.

FLAVOR: Slightly sweet and astringent; they go well on sweet and savory dishes. Sprinkle the petals on your favorite foods to give a pop of color and magic. Or use whole blossoms to decorate a special cake.

Dried rose petals

CHAMOMILE FLOWERS (Matricaria recutita)

A classic and comforting bedtime tea, chamomile is likely one of the first herbs you grew up enjoying. Chamomile is one of our favorite medicinal flowers for adding a bit of whimsy to sweet treats. If growing chamomile in the garden, harvest the blooms often to encourage new blooms so you'll have them all summer long.

FLAVOR: Mildly bitter and sweet, with a hint of apple. They're truly delightful, play well with other aromatic herbs, and are mild enough to enjoy on sweet or savory dishes.

PANSY FLOWERS (Viola x wittrockiana or Viola tricolor)

A classic edible flower that is almost too cute to eat. There are many variations of pansies: blue, yellow, purple, and pink, to name a few. Often you'll see pansies in desserts, but we love adding them to salads, flatbreads, and savory dishes.

FLAVOR: Fresh and mild. Their flavor makes it pretty easy to add their flower power to any dish you want.

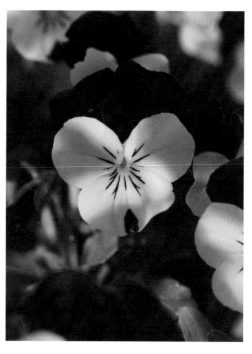

Pansy Flower

Being Mindful in the Kitchen

Through our herbalism practice, we have both developed a deep relationship with the earth. We try our very best to always honor our ecosystems by being resourceful and respectful through our kitchen practice. This means using scraps, reducing trash, composting, buying ethically sourced food (certified organic, fair trade, non-GMO) whenever possible, and holding positive intentions while we create forms of nourishment.

COMPOSTING

In California, we're lucky that composting is done on an industrial level. But we also composted when we lived without this convenience. If you don't have a garden where you can create your own compost, there are fairly cheap composting tumblers and worm bins you can purchase in order to compost right on a small porch. The great thing about the worm bin is that it breaks down kitchen waste into a compost "tea" that can be used as plant food for windowsill herb gardens.

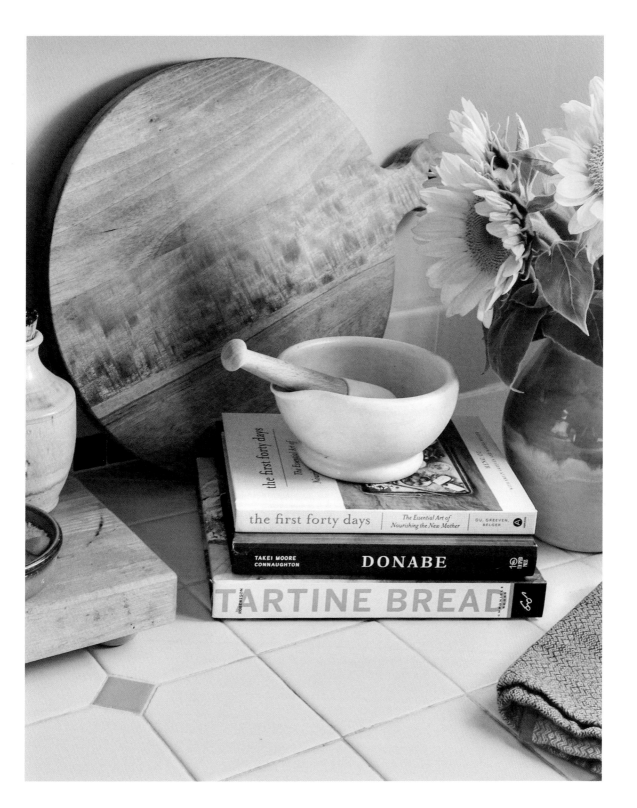

USING SCRAPS

We can reduce most food waste by simply using our scraps. Here are some of our favorite ways to incorporate all the little extras that would otherwise go to waste.

- Freeze leftover soups and sauces.
- Use citrus rinds in cocktails or infuse them into liquor.
- Use onion and garlic skins, the ends of carrots, celery stalks, and leftover pulp from juicing in broths.
- Turn kale, collard, and swiss chard stems into crispy garlic-infused crunchies by pan frying with garlic and ghee.
- Chop up old bread and bake into croutons.
- Create broth out of leftover carcasses or extra bones.
- Use leftover rice to make fried rice.
- Use leftover grains to make sweet or savory porridge or congee.
- Transform wilted herbs or greens into pesto.
- Use leftover nuts and seeds from milk making in baking.
- Infuse vinegar with dried or wilted herbs.
- Create bitters with leftover coffee grounds and rooty bitter herbs.
- Use butter wrappers to grease baking pans.

REDUCING TRASH

While it's not easy to completely cut out trash, there are many ways to avoid it. Here are some thoughts on how to be more mindful when shopping for your kosmic kitchen.

- Use sturdy cooler totes to bring your groceries home. If you do get bags at the store, opt for paper, as you can use these many different ways later on and they're recyclable.
- Bring mesh bags to the store for produce instead of plastic.
- Trade buying salad greens in plastic bins for bulk leafy greens.
- Shop in bulk to avoid using plastic bags. Bring preweighed jars (you can get the empty jars tared with the cashier before shopping) so you can pop them right back on the shelf after purchase or use cotton bulk bags if you need to travel light.
- Use glass reusable containers to marinate meat and veggies. Or use the thick freezer-ready plastic bags, so you can rinse and reuse. Buy durable, reusable, and dishwasher-safe plastic bags online.
- When natural sponges are on their last leg, begin using them for cleaning countertops and stoves instead of dishes. Using dishcloths are great too, since they can be washed and reused.
- If you do end up with plastic to-go containers or grocery items, try your best to reuse them. They can be very useful in which to store chopped veggies or leftovers.

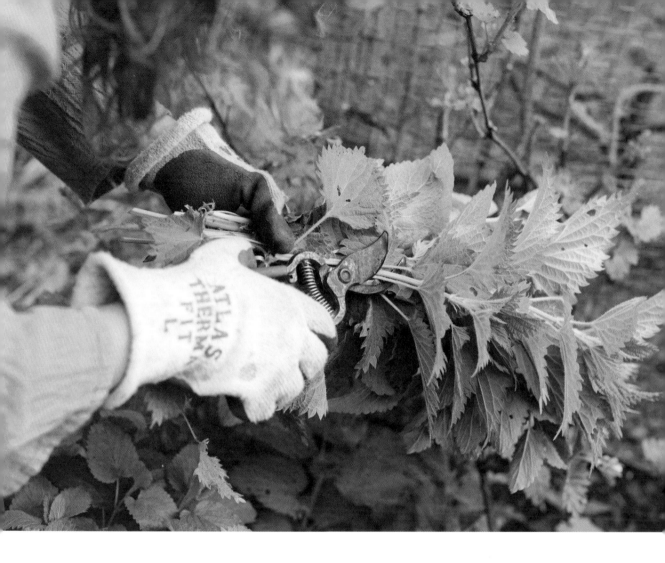

HARVEST RITUALS AND MAKING MEDICINE WITH THE MOON

Whether or not you have a garden, creating a ritual around harvesting or gathering your veggies and herbs is important. If you have a garden, try creating a morning harvest ritual, so that you can collect produce at its prime and create a menu for the day with all your seasonal ingredients top of mind.

If you don't have a garden, try going weekly or biweekly to a local farmers market. Even if you can't afford getting all of your produce there, picking up a few locally grown foods will greatly improve the quality of your meals. The meals you cook will taste better because the ingredients have more intentional energy in them, and you will feel more connected to your community and the seasons. When on a budget, we buy organic produce such as onions, carrots, celery, potatoes, garlic, and citrus from the grocery store and reserve buying eggs, greens, sprouts, and seasonal fruit from our local farmers.

If you feel connected to astrology, you may wish to coordinate making your medicines in accordance with the moon. It's worth noting that the zodiac signs are all ruled by the elements as well. We often make our kitchen medicines—such as Herbal Vinegars (page 104), infused oils, and tinctures—under the darkness of the new moon, as it provides a nourishing and rejuvenating energy as the month following (when the medicine is infusing) is building toward the full moon. You may wish to leave your jars of medicine out overnight to absorb the moonlight as they infuse (*macerate* in herbalism) through a whole moon cycle.

We also love making Herbal Ghee (page 111) and lunar teas using the Cold Water Herbal Infusion method (page 94) during full moons. You'll capture all kinds of different energies depending on the sign the moon is in and the other celestial energies at play.

SETTING INTENTIONS

The energy you bring into the kitchen directly infuses into the food you make. This is why it's so important to set intentions for what you want to bring into meals or remedies and hold those intentions throughout the process of creating. You can do this through chanting, clearing the space through burning herbs, creating a kitchen altar dedicated to your healing intention, playing music that lights you up, dancing while you cook, or whatever stokes your fire!

If your flow gets interrupted, take a moment to pause and clear the space, take some calming herbal tea if you need to, breathe, and restart. These simple resets can really make a difference when you're feeling overwhelmed while cooking. Remember that you're worth the extra time and effort.

Another way to invite intention into your routine is to thank your food before eating. Use this as an opportunity to share your gratitude for the nourishing meal that's in front of you, for the farmers that grew it, for the cook who made it, and for the company of those you're enjoying it with. This practice of gratitude helps ground you back into your body and provides a moment to take a breath so you feel more relaxed before enjoying your meal. As simple as it seems, it has been a ritual we continue to come back to and love to share with friends. Here's a blessing we sing when sitting around the table together that we learned from one of our friends at Herb Pharm. We hope you'll make it your own and sing it with loved ones around your table.

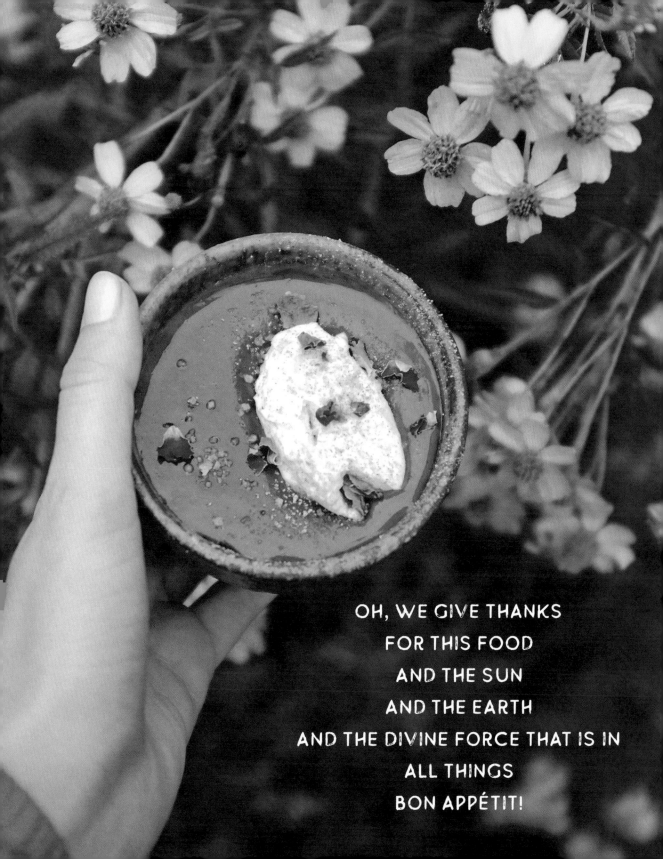

OH, WE GIVE THANKS
FOR THIS FOOD
AND THE SUN
AND THE EARTH
AND THE DIVINE FORCE THAT IS IN
ALL THINGS
BON APPÉTIT!

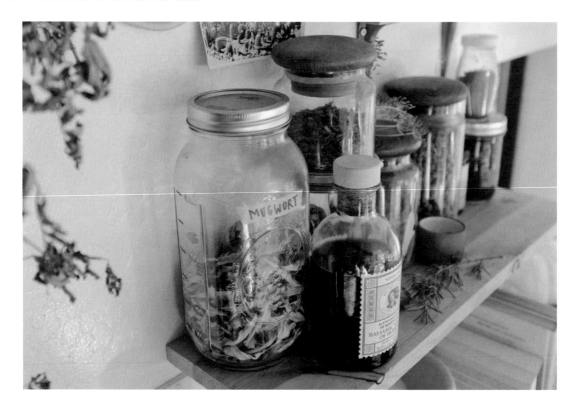

The Magic of Organizing Your Space

Another piece to creating a kosmic kitchen is having an organized space that feels good—space that makes you want to spend time there and calls you to cook. You want your tools and supplies close at hand and ready to go, so you can focus on the creative aspects of nourishing rather than thinking about cleaning up a mess from the night before. Have you ever entered a meditation room or garden that was messy, unorganized, or cluttered? Chances are you haven't. Each object in a space like that has an intention behind why it's there, and the energy of that intention can be felt as soon as you enter the space. Your kosmic kitchen should be the same. Magic happens when we're truly able to shift our perspective of the healing role our kitchen plays in our home. Seeing and treating the kitchen as a sacred space will drastically alter the way you come to your cooking practice each day.

At the same time, we get it: life happens in the kitchen. It isn't always going to be tidy, but we've learned over the years that the more our kitchen feels organized, the more we feel like cooking. And the more we feel like cooking, the easier it is for us to feed ourselves with nourishing herbal foods throughout the week. With the help of a few simple mantras, keeping your kitchen calm, organized, and inviting will feel less like a chore and more like a self-care ritual.

EVERYTHING HAS A PLACE

When our everyday kitchen tools have a home, it makes knowing where to put them or where to find them one less thing to think about. When we haven't created a home for something, we end up not knowing where the heck it is, or spending way too long looking for it. All of this energy distracts us from being in the flow when cooking. Start with the basics: Do your pots and pans have a specific place to live? What about cooking utensils and reusable containers? Everyone's kitchen is different, depending on the size and available storage options, but here are a few of our favorite staples, along with ideas to store them easily.

CAST-IRON SKILLET: The mainstay of our everyday cookware is a cast-iron skillet. It's a universal cooking vessel that, in our kitchen, has seen everything from a summer berry crumble to a quick veggie breakfast scramble. Cast-iron skillets can go from sautéing on the stovetop straight to baking in the oven; they give ingredients a nice sear without drying them out or burning. You can usually find cast-iron skillets at thrift stores for a steal. Look for vintage brands such as Griswold or Wagner that are in good condition—without any cracks or a lot of pitting on the cooking surface. The pitting, or little sand-like bits on the cooking surface, makes it harder to achieve a seasoned nonstick surface that good cast-iron skillets are prized for. Our favorite modern cast-iron brands are Lodge, if you're on a budget, and Le Creuset, if you're looking to invest.

If you don't have a lot of storage, a hanging pot rack is a nice option to get pots, pans, and skillets out of the way but still within reach. Having just one 9-inch cast-iron skillet is all some cooks need. But if you tend to cook a lot or for a large group of people, having a 6-, 9-, and 15-inch cast-iron skillet will be a useful set.

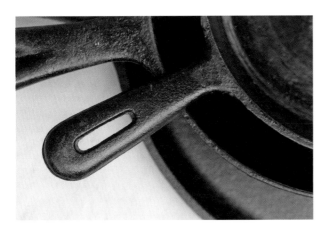

Seasoning a cast-iron skillet is relatively simple and part of ensuring it will last a lifetime. When seasoning, you're preparing the skillet so that it's silky smooth and essentially nonstick, but without the nasty chemicals that coat modern nonstick pans. First, preheat your oven to 350°F. Make sure your cast-iron skillet is clean and dry, and then add about ½ tablespoon of neutral oil, such as flaxseed or sunflower, to the skillet. Using a paper towel or cloth, rub the oil over the entire skillet—even the outside, including the bottom. Once well coated, place the skillet into the oven face down. You can place a sheet of foil on the bottom rack to catch any oil drips. Let the skillet "cook" for an hour, then turn off the oven and

Cast-Iron Skillet

let it cool completely. You should do this when you first get your cast-iron skillet; repeat it every couple of months, or when the surface starts to become less smooth with use.

As for keeping your cast-iron skillet clean between uses, try to remove any leftover bits from cooking with a little coarse salt and water. A good scrub pad or even natural palm scrubbers work best, as they aren't super abrasive and won't leave any scratches. Once your cast-iron skillet is clean, make sure to dry it well by setting it over a low temperature on the stovetop or popping it, skillet side down, in the oven so it can air dry.

DUTCH OVEN: About as versatile as a cast-iron skillet, Dutch ovens are perfect for making bone broths and weeknight soups, simmering a big batch of rooty herbal tea, braising fall-off-the-bone meat, or crafting a one-pot pasta dish. What's great about the Dutch oven is that it holds the heat while cooking and the lid stays on tight, so moisture doesn't escape. This is really the only soup pot you need, and it will last a lifetime. As far as storing goes, ours tends to live right on the stove. A Dutch oven is pretty heavy, so it's best to keep it in an easy-to-reach place or have it out for everyday use. Our favorite brands are Le Creuset, Lodge, and Staub.

CLAY SOUP POT: While a Dutch oven is the only soup pot we need, it's hard to resist earthen cookware. There's something different and more grounding about the way food tastes when it's been cooked in clay. It's a particular kind of alchemy that doesn't happen in other cookware. Whether you're simmering a pot of heirloom beans, making an adaptogenic mushroom broth, or crafting a hearty winter stew, cooking in a clay pot will add an extra layer of comfort.

There are quite a few options in terms of clay cookware. For instance, we love the rich black clay of the La Chamba pots from Colombia. In contrast, we also use traditionally made *donabe* (Japanese earthenware pots), which are made with lighter clay and sometimes glazed white. Whichever clay pot you choose, know that they should only be used on gas stoves, as electric stoves don't distribute heat evenly and can damage the pots. A good way to get around this is to purchase a tabletop butane burner for using a donabe or a heat diffuser for less delicate clay cookware.

We like to keep earthen cookware either on the stove or set out on a shelf or counter to do double duty as decoration. Keeping them visible also makes sure we remember to use them.

SAUCEPAN: A smaller saucepan is great to cook a batch of rice or reheat your daily tea blend or leftover soup. If you don't already have one, find one with a lid, so it's more versatile. We prefer stainless steel or cast-iron saucepans because they're more durable and conduct heat more evenly. Saucepans can usually be kept on the stovetop, if you don't have a lot of storage space, or hung on a pot rack, so they're out of the way. Some of our favorite brands are Le Creuset, All-Clad, and Cuisinart.

TEA KETTLE: A good tea kettle is the mainstay of any herbalist's kitchen. Having one that holds a lot of water and preferably tells you when the water is hot is ideal for making lots of tea throughout the week. This is one kitchen tool you don't want to skimp on. We know from experience that having a reliable tea kettle will save you lots of time and frustration. Look for stainless steel or copper tea kettles when perusing thrift and antique stores, and avoid cheap aluminum ones at all cost.

The Simplex Buckingham, with its classic shape and efficient design, is a top-of-the-line kettle that will last forever. Le Creuset kettles are great too, but they don't make as great of a sound when the water boils. For a pour-over kettle with a slender spout that's perfect for morning coffee or tonics, the Hario has quickly become a classic. Keep your kettle on the stove for everyday use. Just make sure to give it a wipe down every now and then, because they tend to catch a bit of splatter from cooking. An electric kettle can be a great option too. Just make sure it's stainless steel or ceramic, with no plastic parts on the inside.

HERB AND TEA STRAINERS: There are lots of ways to infuse loose tea into water for both infusions and decoctions. We like making herbal infusions in a French press, as it makes the process quick and it's easy to clean up. You can also put herbs in muslin bags when you're infusing heartier herbs into water for a decoction. Stainless steel tea balls work well, and handheld strainers are helpful and can be lined with cheesecloth when straining out small herbs and powders, as mentioned in our Herbal Ghee (page 111) recipe.

BAKING PANS AND BAKING DISHES: Having a couple baking sheets for roasting vegetables, baking galettes, or making cookies and seed crackers comes in handy when you've got a few recipes that need to go in the oven. Baking pans are essential for winter vegetables that become sweeter when roasted and help weeknight meals come together quickly and with minimal cleanup. Look for baking pans that have a little weight to them at kitchen supply shops.

A good rule of thumb to prevent sticking when using baking pans is to line them with parchment paper or silicone baking mats. These options make cleanup a breeze and keep your pans from being stained. Store your baking pans underneath the stove or on their sides in a cupboard so they take up less space and are easy to grab when you need to pop something into the oven.

As far as baking dishes go, we prefer to use ceramic or stoneware dishes. They're usually easy to clean and look nice enough for serving right on the table, so you don't need to put finished food in a serving dish. We find that having a pie dish and a casserole dish is usually enough for the amount of baking we do. Store them near the oven or somewhere you don't have to reach too high or too low, as they can be heavy.

MANDOLIN: Whether you're making matchstick carrots for porridge, tiny radish slices for tacos, or zucchini lasagna, a mandolin will help make the work quick and easy. For the Rainbow Salad with Sweet and Sour Ume Plum Dressing (page 133), use the finest setting to cut your green and red cabbage, or use a thicker setting if you want a more slaw-like crunch. This tool is quite safe when used correctly, though any cook who has been initiated with a battle scar will attest that they can be dangerous when used improperly. We suggest slicing (without an attachment) a few test pieces at the tool's finest setting by sliding the cabbage back and forth across the mandolin and into a large salad bowl. Then taste to assess the texture and adjust the slicing width as desired. You can also use this tool to make rounds, ribbons, and matchsticks with your seasonal veggies. Store in a drawer with the blade facing away from you.

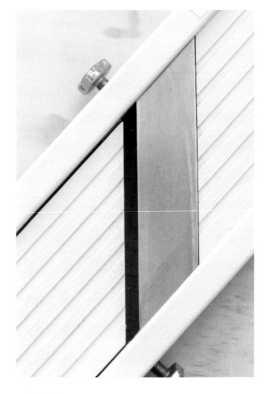

Mandolin

CHEF'S KNIFE: Having a good knife to use daily in the kitchen makes cooking so much more enjoyable. Your cutting and chopping will be more precise, and you're less likely to nick yourself because the knife couldn't cut through something with a dull blade. You don't need to spend a lot of money to get a good knife for everyday cooking. We're lucky to live close to Bernal Cutlery in San Francisco, which carries a great selection of Japanese and French knives (online too) for any budget. When looking for a knife, talk with someone who can show you different types, so you can decide which style is best for you. Remember to keep your knife clean and dry between uses and store in a butcher's block or on a magnetic knife strip for easy access. Treating your knife with care means it will stay sharper longer and stay in good shape.

MORTAR AND PESTLE: Loved by cooks and herbalists alike, a mortar and pestle is a wonderful tool for grinding seeds, splitting spices, pounding fresh ginger, and making a fresh aioli, along with any number of other uses. We prefer to have a ceramic one that's on the smaller side, always out and ready to use. A *suribachi* is a Japanese version with a rough raised pattern on the inside that helps with grinding. Our favorite mortar and pestle is by Milton Brook, but you can find others at most kitchen stores.

MASON JARS: Once you get into a rhythm with your home cooking, you'll never look at glass jars the same. Every jar will look like a home for a precious potion, herbal dressing, or hearty soup. Many of our recipes in this book—including our teas, dressings, and cocktails—are intended to be prepared in mason jars. This makes prep days easy, as your recipes will fit perfectly in these storage containers.

You can save glass jars and lids as you use them or buy a flat or two of mason jars at the local hardware or kitchen store. We suggest getting quart- and pint-sized jars, though all are useful. The mason jars come with metal lids, but you can also invest in durable and reusable plastic or rust-resistant lids to avoid the rust that can occur over time with the metal. We think it's worth noting that before pouring hot tea, broth, or soup into a jar, make sure the jar is at room temperature—not cold—as the hot liquid will likely crack cold glass. Simply run the jar under warm water to get it to room temperature before pouring in the hot water. This little step will save you the headache of having to clean up a big mess from a broken jar.

Throughout the book you will notice larger or batch recipes have serving sizes that indicate the recipe will fill a quart- or pint-size-jar. We suggest purchasing and frequently using these jars so you can easily make and store batches of herbal teas, spices, dressing, broths, and more in your kosmic kitchen.

EVERYTHING YOU NEED IS IN REACH

When organizing your kitchen, think about what you use the most. Everyday staples such as olive oil, sea salt, pepper, wooden spoons, knives, and a good cutting board are basics you might use for just about every meal. Having the essentials within reach of the stove or countertop makes creating a meal easier and more intuitive—it creates a flow when cooking. Knowing where your things are also reduces stress, so you can be more present with your cooking rituals.

Each kitchen has its own set of issues with space, and having a smaller kitchen with less storage can be frustrating. Trust us, we started this work in a rental house that had the tiniest kitchen, with no dishwasher to boot! Kitchens with little to no storage can be a struggle but they can also offer a way to think creatively about efficiency. One way to create more space is by only having what you need. We've all had that feeling of relief after clearing out a ton of things we haven't used or no longer need. Here are some ideas we've implemented over the years that have created more space and beauty in our kitchens.

COUNTERS: Keeping the countertop mostly clear will help when prepping food and cooking. We tend to keep wooden utensils, a bowl of sea salt, olive oil, vinegar, and small spoons for adding spices and herbal powders closest to the stove. Having a stand or cutting board for all these everyday items will save you space and keep everything neatly grouped together.

Keeping kitchen appliances tucked away will save space on your countertop. On the other hand, if there's an appliance you use every day, such as a blender or juicer, keeping that within reach might be a better option than having to constantly put it away and get it out again. Survey your kitchen. What do you have out that is creating less space? Are there things you can store in a drawer or cabinet that would free up counter space?

SHELVES: Having adequate shelving is a lifesaver when it comes to creating efficiency in the kitchen. If you don't have a kitchen with functional cabinetry, open shelving and standing racks are helpful options. Thankfully, they're usually inexpensive to install and allow you to easily see what you have. We like to keep an herb shelf in the forefront of our kitchen to store daily adaptogenic powders, dried

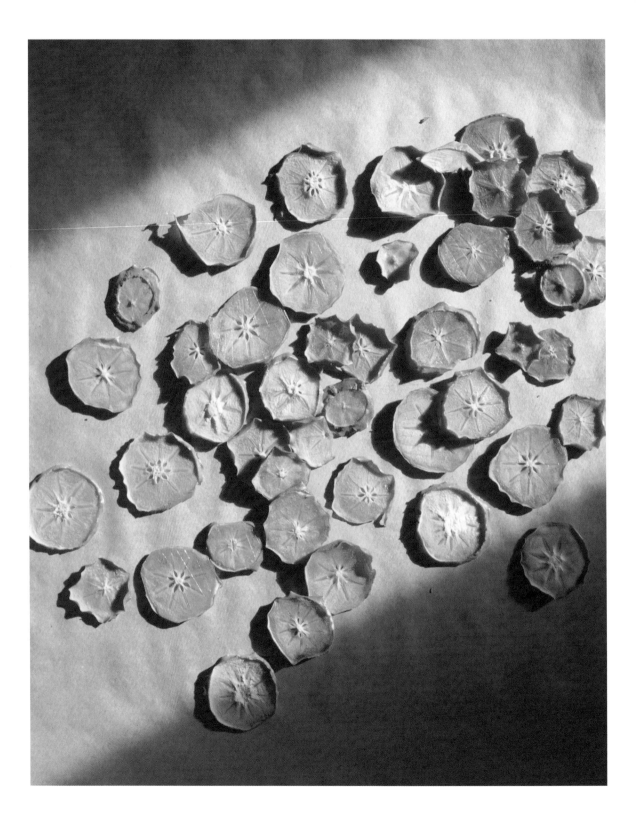

spices, herbal sprinkles, salts, and specialty ingredients we might forget to use if they were tucked away. Keeping herbs sealed in glass jars and out of direct sunlight will keep them fresher longer and help maintain their potency. Clear jars are nice for spices, since their color and texture will help you discern one from another. If you prefer amber or blue jars, we recommend creating labels with washi tape and a permanent marker.

For pantry and cabinet shelves, mason jars and labels with washi tape will come in handy too. You can easily see what you have and know when you need to restock. You can even take your jars to the bulk aisle, already marked with the tare weight at the bottom, to reduce using plastic packaging. Usually, we keep our everyday dry goods in a cabinet or on a shelf within reach of our prep space. Store everything else in a pantry or cabinet with the labels facing out. Flat-bottomed woven baskets can be helpful to group like ingredients together on shelves. For instance, create a baking basket, a grains basket, a legume basket, a seeds and nuts basket; or group together any similar containers or bags of ingredients you use in tandem, so you can locate them more easily.

CLEAN AS YOU GO SO THERE'S NO STRESS LATER

Our foundation for prepping nourishing meals is this mantra: Clean as you go. We're not perfect when it comes to cleaning, but when we take a few extra minutes to clean as we go, it saves us a lot of time and stress. This can be as simple as cleaning up scraps and wiping down your cutting board after chopping vegetables. Rinsing prep dishes before serving a meal is helpful too. That way when you're done enjoying your meal, you only need to wash the dishes you ate from and the pot you cooked in, rather than a whole stack. Everyone gets into their own rhythm with this, but next time you cook, see how it feels to clean as you go.

And cleaning doesn't have to feel like a chore, especially if you're using products that are gentle and have a pleasing aroma. Most cleaning products you find in the store labeled "natural" truly aren't and often have toxic artificial fragrances. Instead, distilled vinegar, Dr. Bronner's all-purpose soap, baking soda, and Citra Solv are our go-to multipurpose ingredients, and we use them to make inexpensive and nontoxic cleaning supplies.

We dilute Dr. Bronner's soap with a little water in a jar with a pump and use it for everyday dish soap. You can also make a solution of 1 part distilled white vinegar with 1 part water and a few drops of lavender essential oil to use as an all-purpose cleaner in a spray bottle. This is an effective multipurpose cleaner for countertops, floors, and other surfaces (such as the inside of your refrigerator). Get creative and simplify the products you use. Baking soda is great when you need a gentle abrasive to get grime from a cast-iron skillet or to clean grout. What we use to clean after we cook is just as important as what we're putting in our bodies to nourish ourselves.

Prepping for a Nourishing Week

We know life is busy. It's hard enough sometimes to figure out what to make for dinner, let alone have the time to go shopping or feel relaxed enough to actually cook. This is where the magical art of prepping comes in to give your week a sense of ease while ensuring you'll have something nourishing on hand when you get home from a busy day. Now, don't let this sound like yet another thing to tack on to your to do list. Instead, think of it as your support system.

The way we prep for the week starts by looking at the calendar. This gives us a better sense of when we will be home for dinner and which days we might have a full schedule with no time to cook. Then we plan out the week's meals and remedies based on how much we have going on. We use Sunday to take stock of what we have in the fridge and go shopping for fresh ingredients. Sunday (or whatever your prep day might be) is also a great time to prep simple things that you'll use all week, to save time during the week.

To keep things streamlined, we stick to two breakfast options and a few lunch and dinner options per week. This doesn't mean we eat the same thing all the time, but by using similar ingredients in different preparations throughout the week, we cut down on prepping and cooking. Here are a few tips to create a prep day each week and stay organized throughout the week.

PREP AND STORE PRODUCE

After purchasing your produce for the week, wash, dry, chop, and store as much as you can neatly fit in your refrigerator. Having reusable cloth produce bags will make storing things easier and reduce the amount of plastic you use when shopping. For dark leafy greens and lettuces, remove the stems and chop or tear the greens into bite-sized pieces. We love to chop up the stems to add to soups, stews, or quick stir-fries. Store in cloth bags or wrapped in moist kitchen cloths.

For carrots, beets, sweet potatoes, and other root vegetables, wash well to remove excess soil and chop to desired sizes for meals during the week. To get the most out of your vegetables, save any green tops to use in Wild Weeds Pesto (see page 102). Store vegetables in tightly sealed glass reusable containers.

Showcase fresh herbs on the kitchen counter by simply cutting off a bit of the bottom of the stems for freshness and placing in a small glass or jar with water. Think of it as an herbal kitchen bouquet. This way, the herbs will always be in view and will inspire fresh flavors for your recipes.

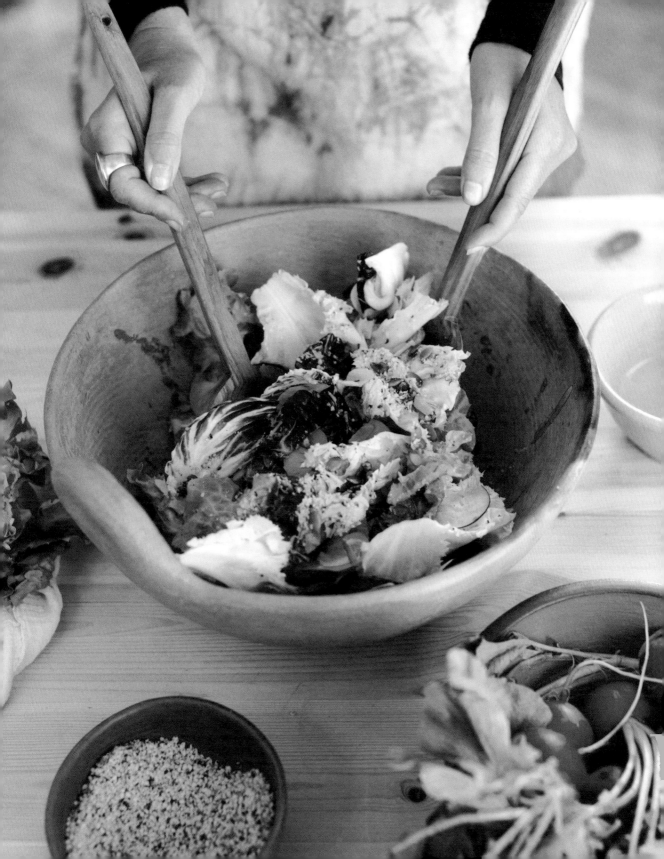

SOAK AND SPROUT GRAINS, SEEDS, LEGUMES, AND NUTS

Take a look at your meals for the week. What will you need to soak overnight before cooking? Make a note of this on your phone or on a list that you can stick on your refrigerator, so you've a game plan for the day. We like to begin soaking the next day's grains or legumes as we clean up from dinner. That way when we wake up, we can strain and rinse them or put them on to cook so they're ready to enjoy when we get home for dinner.

SOAKING GRAINS: Soaking grains, or prefermenting, is a practice held by all of our ancestors. It's ancient, intuitive, and necessary to get the most out of food. Grains are seeds that store nutrients and life until they're ready to meet the world in an optimal environment. Since plants are so smart, they use certain chemicals, such as phytic acid, to prevent sprouting in an unfavorable environment where they won't be able to grow into maturity. According to food activist and fermentation revivalist Sandor Katz in his book *The Art of Fermentation*, "Phytic acid reduces the availability of minerals not only in the food that contains phytic acid, but also in other foods being digested at the same time." By soaking your grains, you're awakening the grains—transforming and neutralizing the harmful effects of phytic acid and increasing the bioavailability of other nutrients.

Luckily, soaking grains is super easy and takes less than thirty seconds of prep time. Just put the desired amount of grain you want to cook in a bowl and cover completely with warm water. Pour in 1 to 2 tablespoons of some live active cultures, such as whey, buttermilk, yogurt, apple cider vinegar, or lemon juice. It's also important to use filtered water rather than tap, since the chlorine in most municipal water systems can hinder the beneficial bacteria and fungi from being able to predigest grains.

Leave the bowl on the kitchen counter covered with a towel for at least 1 hour but preferably overnight. In the morning, rinse and strain the grains with a mesh colander. If you forget to soak overnight, allowing the grains to soak in water, even if only for 1 hour, helps to revive the surface of each grain with the naturally present fungi and bacteria responsible for the fermentation. Keep in mind that soaking reduces the cook time and the amount of water you need to cook with. We usually reduce the water by ¼ cup and cook 5 to 10 minutes less, depending on the grain.

Cooking tip: An easy way to cook soaked rice, quinoa, or millet without ever burning it is to bring it to a boil while covered, then turn off the heat. Keep covered for 10 minutes or so, then remove the lid and fluff the grain with a fork. Cooks perfectly every time.

SPROUTING SEEDS AND LEGUMES: Sprouts are basically baby plants—new life budding into the world. All this new energy makes for a vital food that has already been predigested for you through the germination process. Sprouting increases the vitamin (especially vitamin C) and enzyme content dramatically. It also allows for better assimilation and metabolization of nutrients, because it neutralizes

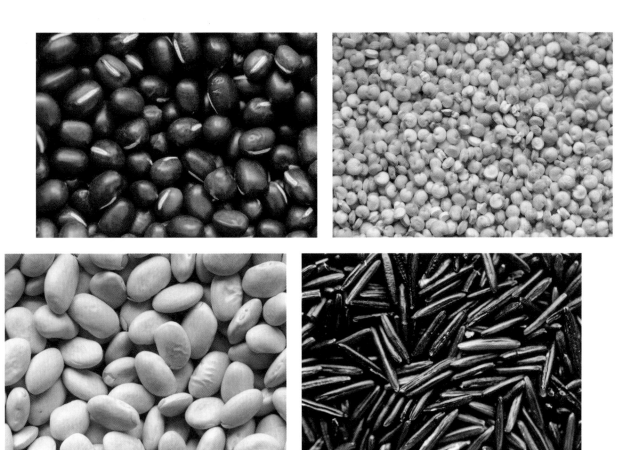

the phytic acid. Sprouting is simple, inexpensive, and ensures you're getting the freshest sprouts out there, whereas store-bought sprouts can be expensive and less than fresh.

We like to use a mason jar to sprout. The first step to sprouting grains and legumes is to soak them in water overnight. Sprouting, or germination, requires water and oxygen. Sprouting won't occur during the soaking process because not enough oxygen will be present.

Simply fill the jar a quarter of the way full of your seed or legume of choice, cover them with water, and let them soak overnight with either a screen lid or a piece of cheesecloth secured with a rubber band. In the morning, strain and rinse the seeds in the jar, letting the excess water drain out by placing the jar in a bowl at an angle or on your dish rack. The jar should have some space between the lid and the bottom of the bowl because you don't want the sprouts sitting in excess water. Again, it's important to use filtered water rather than tap, since the chlorine in most municipal water can prevent sprouts from forming.

Repeat the rinse in the evening and continue to keep the sprouts moist by rinsing twice a day. Depending on the hardiness of the seed and the temperature of your home, it will take anywhere from 3 to 5 days for the seeds or legumes to sprout little tails.

SPROUTING NUTS: To sprout nuts such as almonds, put 1 cup of nuts in a quart-sized mason jar, cover with 3 cups of warm water, and stir in 1 teaspoon sea salt (instead of the acid used for sprouting grains). Cover with a lid and let sit on the counter overnight. Walnuts and pecans, which have been removed from their shells, can't be sprouted. However, soaking these types of nuts overnight in warm sea salt water will help neutralize the phytic acid. Use unchlorinated water for best results, as chlorine can inhibit sprout formation. To continue to sprout the soaked nuts, strain out the water, give them a rinse, and return them to the jar. Cover the top with cheesecloth or a sprouting screen (found at most hardware stores) and leave for the day in a sunny windowsill. Repeat this process of soaking, rinsing, and letting the nuts sit in the sun, until tiny tails or sprouts appear throughout the nuts.

WHAT TO DO WITH SOAKED AND SPROUTED NUTS AND SEEDS

You can keep soaked nuts in the fridge as a snack; we've found their flavor is much sweeter after soaking. In a glass jar with a tight-fitting lid, they will last in the fridge for up to 1 week. If you want your nuts to keep a crunchy consistency, use a dehydrator for 8 to 12 hours, and then we suggest storing them in the freezer. (Check your specific dehydrator for temperatures for nuts and seeds.)

You can also make fresh plant milks with the soaked-sprouted nuts and seeds. Some of our favorite nuts and seeds to use are pumpkin, sunflower, sesame, almond, and cashew. In general, the ratio for a creamy milk is 1 part nuts or seeds to 4 parts water. Add the nuts, water, a pinch of sea salt, a date or two, and a teaspoon of vanilla extract to a high-powered blender. Blend until smooth and strain through a nut milk bag or a tight mesh strainer. Store the milk in a glass mason jar with a tight-fitting lid in the fridge. It will keep for 3 to 5 days, and you can use it in coffee, tea, smoothies, or whatever else you dream up.

Keep in mind that sprouted foods are cooling in nature. They're great to use during the warmer months of spring and summer. If your constitution tends to be on the cooler end of the spectrum, you can always lightly sauté or steam sprouts or add them to soups and stews without altering their healing benefits.

TOASTED NUTS AND SEEDS

Toasted nuts and seeds are a kosmic kitchen staple. We usually make a big batch on Sunday so we have them handy to garnish our veggies, salads, and porridges throughout the week. Use a cast-iron skillet and set the temperature on low to medium heat. Add a few pinches of salt or whatever seasonal spices you want to incorporate. Then add the nuts or seeds and stir them occasionally so they're evenly toasted. They should be ready in just a few minutes. For seeds, you will know they're ready because some of them will begin to pop and smell nutty. Another way to tell they're ready is by the color: you want both sides to reach a golden-brown hue.

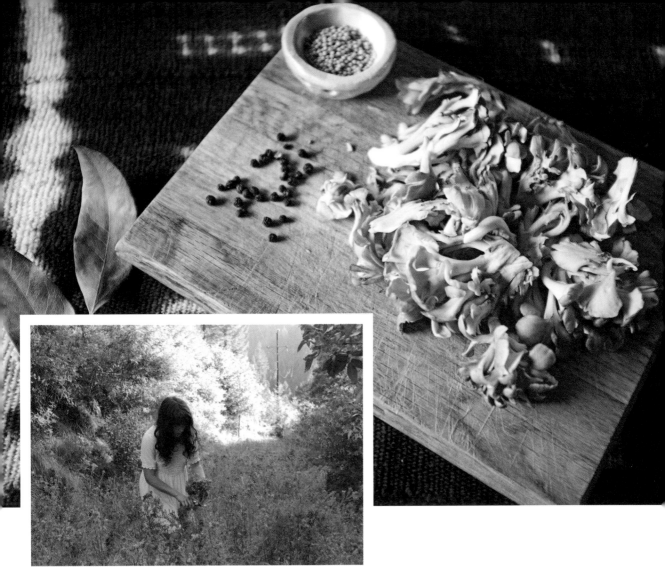

MAKING YOUR MEDICINES

We'll go over these recipes in the next section, as they take only minutes to make and provide your weekly meals with extra-special nourishing flavors. Whether it's Wild Weeds Pesto (page 102), herbal dips or sauces, Herbal Honey (page 108), Herbal Dressings (page 105), Herbal Power Bites (page 114), or Herbal Ghee (page 111), make as many of your extras as you can on your prep day so there's less to do throughout the week. Just assess what you already have in the fridge and choose a few to make ahead of time, so you can restock prior to shopping.

This is also a great time to create a seasonal tea blend for the upcoming week. Or if you're including tinctures in your routine, pull out the medicines you're working with and keep them somewhere you will see them, to ensure you use them each day.

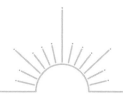

Herbal Preps and Extras

BECAUSE WE RELY ON HOME COOKING AS THE backbone of our wellness practice, our kosmic kitchen shelves are filled with mason jars full of dried goods such as grains, legumes, nuts, seeds, dried fruits, dried herbs, seaweeds, oils, salts, herbs, and spices—ingredients that require the alchemy of cooking to come alive. Creating herbal preps and adding in extras such as medicinal seaweed and high-quality sea salts will add so much flavor and medicine to your week of meals. If you make super-simple things each day, having an herbal extra on hand is a great way to not only add delicious flavors but also make sure you're getting medicinal herbs on your plate. Having ready-made herbal foods allows us to walk into the kitchen knowing a nourishing meal or a beverage will only take a few minutes to make.

These herbal preps can also be used in a variety of ways. For instance, our Tulsi Pesto (page 169) can be used as a dressing or dip, and our Adaptogenic Ginger Maca Miso Dressing (page 106) can be used on salads, over roasted veggies, or with soba noodles. Once you get into a routine of preparing your favorites each week, you won't be able to imagine your kitchen without them. We'll show you how to create your own herbal extras that allow you to use the herbs and flavors most balancing to your dosha and nourish you throughout the seasons.

INFUSIONS

Herbal infusions are an easy and effective way to enjoy medicinal herbs, since many herbal properties are extracted well in water. The ritual of making infusions, or "herbal tea," is one of our favorite ways to take a few moments to ground ourselves during the day. Though true tea—green, white, and black—is made from the *Camellia sinensis* plant, herbal infusions refer to making tea with more delicate parts of plants, such as the leaves and flowers.

To get the full therapeutic properties from herbs that support the whole body, sipping 3 to 4 cups of tea a day is ideal. To make this process

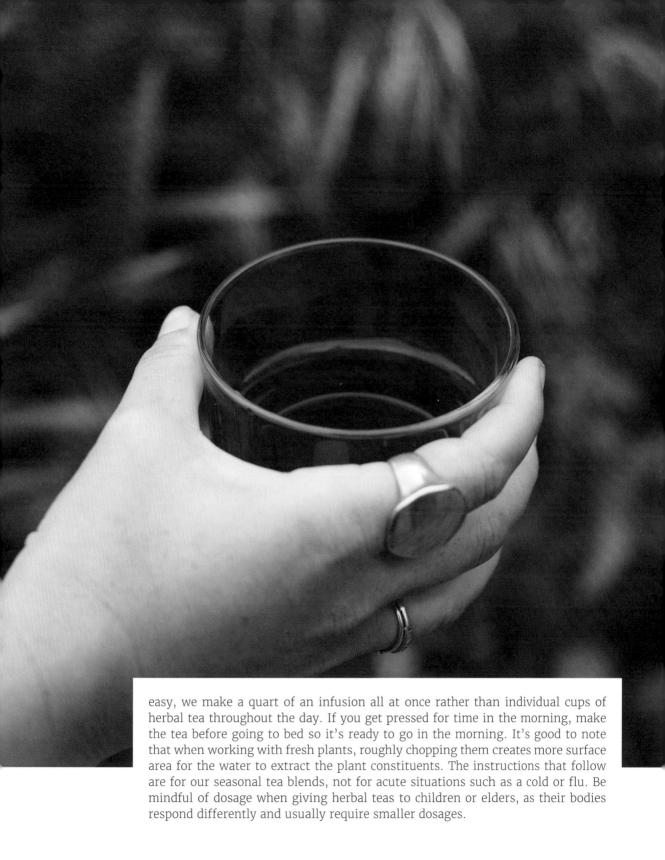

easy, we make a quart of an infusion all at once rather than individual cups of herbal tea throughout the day. If you get pressed for time in the morning, make the tea before going to bed so it's ready to go in the morning. It's good to note that when working with fresh plants, roughly chopping them creates more surface area for the water to extract the plant constituents. The instructions that follow are for our seasonal tea blends, not for acute situations such as a cold or flu. Be mindful of dosage when giving herbal teas to children or elders, as their bodies respond differently and usually require smaller dosages.

Hot Water Herbal Infusions

This method is best for plant parts that are high in tannins and essential oils such as the aerial and more delicate parts of plants, which means the aboveground portions, such as leaves, flowers, and some seeds. **FILLS 1 QUART-SIZED JAR**

2 tablespoons cut and sifted, dried herbs or ½ cup fresh herbs, chopped

1 quart water, boiled

Raw local honey, optional

+ NOTE: There are a few things to note here when using a glass mason jar. First, make sure the jar is room temperature—not cold—as the hot water will likely crack cold glass. Simply run the jar under warm water to get it to room temperature before pouring in the hot water.

In a quart-sized mason jar, add your herbs, then pour the boiled water over, making sure to saturate the herbs. Cover lightly with a lid or saucer to trap the beneficial essential oils and let it steep for 15 to 30 minutes or overnight. The longer the mixture infuses, the more potent (and often bitter) it will become. Use a small mesh strainer or French press to strain out the herbs and compost or discard. Pour the infusion into another quart-sized jar. Lightly sweeten with honey, if you'd like, or enjoy as is throughout the day. If not using immediately, let cool and store in the fridge for up to 2 days. ■

Cold Water Herbal Infusions

Cold water infusions are ideal for plants that are high in polysaccharides and have mucilage, such as marshmallow, slippery elm, or licorice. It's also a great method for vitamin- and mineral-rich herbs such as rose hips and nettle, because when you heat these herbs you can lose some of their beneficial nutrients. Cold water infusion is a wonderful way to get the soothing and cooling properties of these plants and one of our favorite preparations during the hottest months of the year for a refreshing herbal beverage. Just make sure to refrigerate the infusion if you're not using it immediately, to keep it fresh.

FILLS 1 QUART-SIZED JAR

2 tablespoon cut and sifted, dried   1 quart cool water
herbs or ½ cup fresh herbs, chopped

Place your herbs in a muslin bag and bundle tightly. Fill your quart-sized mason jar with water, leaving a few inches from the top. Moisten the herbs with a little water, then submerge them in the quart jar, letting the excess string from the muslin bag hang over the edge. Screw on the lid so that the muslin bag is floating, rather than sinking to the bottom. This suspension helps circulate fresh water to the herbs. Let the infusion sit overnight or for about 8 hours, either on the counter or in the fridge. Remove the muslin bag and discard or compost the herbs. Enjoy throughout the day or store in the fridge for up to 2 days. ■

Making a Single Cup of Tea

While we rarely make a single cup of tea, other than using tea bags when traveling, it's good to know how to make a proper herbal infusion for acute situations. Using herbal tea when sick with a cold, a flu, or digestive upset can be really helpful and soothing. We often use 1 teaspoon to 1 tablespoon of dried herbs, depending on the cut we've purchased. The finer the cut, the less you need to use. Plus, we often make more than 8 ounces and love a strong brew made with the restorative herbs, which are what we mainly use throughout this book.

1 teaspoon to 1 tablespoon cut and   1 cup hot water
sifted, dried herbs or 2 tablespoons
fresh herbs, chopped

Place your herbs in a small French press or teapot/teacup with mesh strainer and pour the hot water over. Cover with a top and let steep for 8 to 15 minutes. Strain out the herbs and compost or discard. Pour the tea into your favorite teacup or mug and enjoy. ■

Decoctions

In order to make an herbal drink with hardier parts of plants—such as the bark, roots, dried berries, or seeds—the plant parts must be simmered or decocted in water to extract, rather than just steeping. It's helpful to think about what plant parts you're using in a formula, so the preparation makes sense for the plants in the mix. If you have a blend that you're creating with leaves and flowers along with roots and barks, think about ways to make the formula with only plants that need to be decocted, so you don't lose any of the precious properties from the more delicate plants that should be infused instead. Or, if there's a mix of roots and barks, simply infuse the blend for a bit longer, and opt for a finer cut for best extraction.

Decoctions are wonderful for rich, rooty plants such as dandelion root, burdock, ashwagandha, licorice root, and reishi. Whole spices also do well in decoctions, as they tend to be hardier and release more flavor in a longer brew.

FILLS 1 QUART-SIZED JAR

Dried roots, barks, berries, and seeds

1 quart water, boiled

2 to 3 tablespoons cut and sifted, dried herbs

Raw local honey to taste, optional

In a saucepan, add your herbs and water and bring to a simmer, covered. Keeping the pot covered, let the herbs decoct on a low simmer for 20 to 45 minutes. The longer it brews, the stronger the tea will be. Strain out the herbs using a mesh strainer or French press and compost or discard. If desired, sweeten with honey, since a lot of roots and seeds can be on the bitter side. Cool and store the decoction in a mason jar in the fridge for up to 2 days. ■

SEAWEEDS

In general, all seaweeds contain high amounts of iodine, making seaweed a great supplement for those who want to support healthy thyroid function. If you have a thyroid disorder, consult your practitioner on dose and proper use as an everyday supplement, as too much iodine can also cause problems.

It's also important to source seaweed from a reputable source, as environmental toxins can accumulate in these sea vegetables, and to support sustainable harvest practices. Learn more by going to our buying guide on page 251.

DULSE: A red algae that is harvested from the Pacific and Atlantic Oceans, dulse has been collected for thousands of years and used in European and Asian seaside cuisines for its unique umami flavor and rich nutritional value. It's full of vitamins and minerals and packs a hefty amount of protein and fiber. The Irish call it *dillisk* and commonly pair it with butter, adding it into baked breads and soups. We love sprinkling it over our food to get in some extra vitamin C and iodine for thyroid support.

KOMBU: Famously known to make beans more digestible, kombu is a staple in macrobiotic diets. We use this brown algae when cooking beans and in mineral-rich broths. Simply add in one strip to the pot and this enzyme-rich seaweed will break down the bean's complex sugars. It's also the main ingredient in dashi, a staple umami broth that is the base flavor in most Japanese cooking. See our Nourishing Nettle Soup with White Beans and Shiitakes (page 134) and Mineral-Rich Seaweed and Mushroom Broth (page 113).

NORI: Commonly eaten as a snack and used as the wrapping for sushi, this red algae is a traditional staple in Japan. Unlike other seaweeds, nori is largely cultivated for commerce due to advanced farming innovations, making it more widely available. It's rich in vitamins A and C, riboflavin, folate, and iodine. We buy it in dried sheets to make veggie sushi wraps in the warmer seasons or toasted and crushed as a garnish on miso soup and noodles. See our Black Sesame Seed and Seaweed Gomasio on page 101.

SALTS

We can't live without salt. Not only is it essential to flavor our meals but also to our body's ability to function. The story of how these ocean and river salt crystals form is something magical. When the chloride and sodium molecules of the water make their journey to the shore, they react with the magnesium and potassium molecules of the earth, and in that moment forms the edible crystal we know as salt. Table salt, which is stripped of all its precious minerals, is actually dehydrating to the body and should be avoided.

When dissolved in water, salt creates compounds called electrolytes that have an ionic charge, which conducts energy and allows our cells to communicate. Electrolytes are an essential part of how our cells function. They're crucial to how our kidneys function and how well they assimilate water for hydration. In the body, electrolytes regulate nerve and muscle function and acidity and fluid levels, and they determine how hydrated we are.

You can get electrolytes by adding natural salt (not table salt) to your water or using salt as a seasoning on your food. We use about 1/4 to 1/2 teaspoon in a 16-ounce (or more) ceramic or glass water bottle and sip slowly throughout the day to stay hydrated. Try adding salt to your water to taste. Everyone is different. It should taste slightly saline but not like ocean water. Start on the lower end of dosage if you're sensitive, and see how your body reacts. Too much salt can act as a purgative or laxative, which is not the goal here. Add salt to water without using a metal spoon or leaving metal in the glass, as metal can deionize electrolytes. It's also best to add salt to food after cooking if using metal pans. It's important not to chug, as lots of salt at once can cause nausea for those new to the practice.

Being more conscious about salt has been incredibly transformative in how hydrated we are. Instead of guzzling down jars and jars of water, we're much more hydrated from less water and find we're not depleting our systems of valuable electrolytes. Remember, when we aren't hydrated, we're running dry and this can result in irritability, anxiety, or dry skin. Try adding some salt to your water in the morning and see how you feel throughout the day. Did you feel more hydrated? Less irritated? More energized? Stick with this for a week or more to really get a sense of how hydrated you feel.

There are many types of salts from all over the world, and each has their own unique qualities based on the conditions from which they're harvested. To keep it simple, the energetics of salt can be seen in their color. Cooling salts are lighter in color; warming salts are darker in color. Salts can come in many textures from fine to fractal pyramids. Below are a few of our favorites that can be easily found online or in specialty stores.

ATLANTIC GRAY SEA SALT: This is our go-to salt for everyday seasoning and adding to water. It's slightly wet to the touch and hydrating in nature, which makes it beneficial to the kidneys. Its gray color indicates it's high in magnesium and cooling.

FRENCH GRAY SEA SALT (SEL GRIS): One of the most iconic artisanal French salts, *sel gris* is as beautiful as it is delicious. This crunchy sea salt is lovely sprinkled over soups, salads, roasted vegetables, and chocolate. Its gray color indicates that it's high in magnesium and energetically cooling in nature.

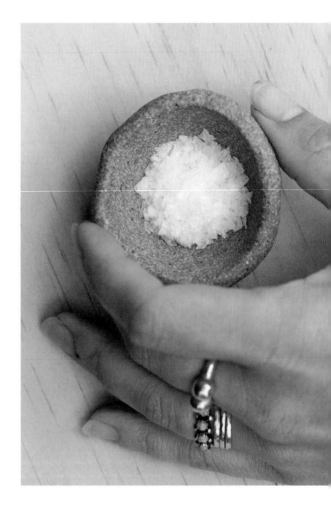

CYPRUS FLAKE SALT: Another beautiful finishing salt, this flake salt is known for its unique crystalline pyramid shape and nice crunch. Its pearly white color signifies richness in potassium and cooling nature. We love to sprinkle it over fresh salads to add the perfect hint of flavor.

Kosmic Kurry Spice Blend

This is our take on a spice blend that has a somewhat complicated history. Curry, indicative of Indian food and flavors, usually brings to mind a medley of warming spices that can be found packaged in the spice aisle. Curry is also a plant with aromatic leaves with a similar scent to a blend of Eastern spices. It's believed that curry powder evolved as a way for British spice traders to more easily ship and store the prized herbs sought from India back to England. The word *curry* comes from the Tamil word *kari*, which means "to blacken" or "to season." Colonizers tend to generalize complex and ancient food ways, thus curry came to be known as a packaged spice rather than distinct dishes enjoyed across India, Thailand, Malaysia, Sri Lanka, Indonesia, and many places in between. In the West, we've come to know curry as a spiced sauce served with rice and vegetables or meat. While this meaning of curry has taken hold and we recognize its history, our version is a nod to the healing properties of the spices in the blend.

Make enough to fill a spice jar or a larger jar if you know you'll go through a bigger batch. We provide the ratios we use below, but feel free to experiment by adding in more or less of the flavors you love. Adaptogens pair well in this blend, as certain ones, such as ashwagandha, can have a strong flavor. A "part" simply means a ratio, so it's equivalent to 1 teaspoon, 1 tablespoon, 1 ounce, or even 1 cup. ADAPTABLE

1 part ground turmeric

1/4 part ground cinnamon

1/4 part ground cardamom

1/4 part ground cumin

1/4 part ground coriander

1/4 part whole fennel seeds

1/4 part powdered adaptogens such as ashwagandha, maca, or shatavari

In a mixing bowl, mix all of the spices together with a spoon until combined. Store in a jar with a tight lid or in a spice jar. Keep out of direct sunlight, and use within 6 months to 1 year. ■

Kitchari Blend

Kitchari, or *khichuri*, is a warming and comforting traditional dish of the subcontinent of India, made with split dahl, mung beans, lentils or other quick-cooking pulses, rice, and spices. In Ayurveda, you'll likely see kitchari during times when the digestive system needs a break to facilitate healing in the body. Because the combination of rice and lentils makes kitchari a complete protein, the body receives nourishment without having to expend a lot of energy breaking down and assimilating complex foods.

The spices used in kitchari also depend on who's making it and where they are. While the history of kitchari is deep and varies from place to place, we like to make a simple version adopted from our favorite Ayurvedic author, Dr. Vasant Lad. By having a ready-made kitchari spice blend on hand, you'll have one less step when creating this healing dish. MAKES ABOUT ½ CUP

2 tablespoons ground turmeric

2 tablespoons whole fennel seeds

2 tablespoons whole coriander seeds

2 tablespoons whole cumin seeds

2 tablespoons whole mustard seeds

In a small bowl, mix all the spices together with a spoon until combined. Store in a small jar with a tight lid or double the quantity and divide among spice jars to share with friends. ■

THE HERBS USED IN KITCHARI ALSO PLAY IMPORTANT ROLES IN SUPPORTING THE BODY. HERE ARE A FEW OF THEM AND THEIR BENEFITS.

TURMERIC: *This herb helps strengthen the digestion and improve intestinal flora. Energetically, it's warming, blood purifying, and stimulating for the formation of new blood tissues. It also promotes proper metabolism, correcting both excesses and deficiencies.*

FENNEL SEEDS: *One of the best herbs for digestion and digestive weakness in children or the elderly. Fennel also calms the nerves and promotes mental alertness.*

CORIANDER: *This herb increases digestion and absorption of nutrients. It's used with cumin and fennel to promote the assimilation of other herbs.*

CUMIN: *A carminative with bitter and pungent flavors, cumin helps stimulate the digestive system and ease intestinal discomfort. It also helps gently remove toxins from the system.*

MUSTARD SEEDS: *Warming and pungent, mustard seeds help stimulate digestion, making them an ally for those who tend to run cold. They add a lovely texture and pop of color to many dishes. Try them sautéed in ghee to bring out their aroma. Just make sure the pan lid is close at hand, so they don't scatter all over the kitchen as they begin to pop.*

Black Sesame Seed and Seaweed Gomasio

Gomasio is a sesame seed and sea salt condiment first introduced to us at Tassajara Zen Mountain Center. There was a heaping bowl of gomasio served with every meal to sprinkle on grains, vegetables, or fresh greens. This salty, nutty seasoning adds a delightful crunch we can't seem to get enough of. Perhaps you've seen gomasio as part of the Japanese macrobiotic diet. You can keep this gomasio recipe simple by just roasting the sesame seeds and salt, or add in toasted seaweed, such as nori, for more minerals. The key here is grinding the seeds to break them down in order to digest them. We like to make a batch that will last us for a week or more. MAKES ABOUT 2 CUPS

1 cup white sesame seeds

1 cup black sesame seeds

2 teaspoons fine sea salt

1 sheet dried nori, torn into 1-inch pieces, optional

Preheat the oven to 350°F and line a baking sheet with parchment paper. In a bowl, toss the sesame seeds, sea salt, and nori together to mix. Spread the mixture onto the prepared baking sheet and toast for 5 to 7 minutes. Halfway through the roasting time, rotate the baking sheet and stir the mixture to prevent the seeds on the edge from getting too toasted. Once toasted and fragrant, remove the sheet from the oven to cool. Working in ¼-cup batches, add the toasted mixture to a mortar and pestle or suribachi and grind the seeds and nori to your liking. We prefer a ratio of about ½ ground seeds to ½ whole seeds. Store in a mason jar with a tight-fitting lid in the fridge to keep the seeds fresh for up to 6 months. ∎

Wild Weeds Pesto

A classic staple in many herbalists' kitchens, there's truly nothing like the taste of freshly made herbal pesto with wild weeds from the garden. Traditionally pesto is made with pine nuts, garlic, parmesan cheese, olive oil, and fresh sweet basil and is either chopped by hand or macerated with a mortar and pestle. It's an addictive sauce that accompanies many savory dishes. Our version consists of the same basic principles: fatty nuts or seeds, good olive oil, garlic, and fresh herbs. We've been known to add a little parmesan into our pesto, but usually it's dairy free, as that makes a lighter pesto and is an easy option for inclusive cooking.

There are a lot of wild weeds growing around us or in the garden. Wild herbs and greens offer us a wider spectrum of nutrients that we can't get in produce we find in the grocery store. Making a wild weeds pesto from the garden is a wonderful way to incorporate these humble and often overlooked allies.

This recipe can be adapted with a variety of fresh medicinal herbs throughout the seasons. In late winter and early spring there's always an abundance of chickweed—a bright green, low-growing, sweet plant with tiny white flowers. Its slightly bitter flavor indicates its ability to support the lymphatic system and liver after the cold and stagnant winter season. During the summer, nettle is the star, offering an abundance of vitamins and minerals while also contributing its slightly bitter and cooling flavor. In the fall, dandelion greens and dark leafy greens lend themselves to support our digestive system with their slightly bitter flavor, encouraging the liver and gallbladder to process fats and excess heat. The winter months are a great time to add warming herbs and flavors to your pesto. Think extra garlic, fresh ginger, and even leeks to warm up the flavor profile and help support healthy circulation.

Some of our favorite ways to enjoy this pesto are by adding a dollop to runny eggs in the morning, mixing it into rice for a side dish, spooning it on top of a creamy pumpkin soup, or thinning it down with olive oil and lemon juice for a salad dressing. MAKES ABOUT 2 CUPS

2 garlic cloves, smashed

1 cup raw pumpkin seeds

¼ to ½ teaspoon sea salt

4 cups or two big handfuls of fresh herbs or greens (tulsi, lemon balm, cilantro, parsley, or chickweed)

1 cup olive oil

Juice of 1 lemon

In a food processor, combine garlic, pumpkin seeds, and sea salt. Pulse a few times until the seeds break down to a coarse texture. For a creamier pesto, pulse the pumpkin seeds into a finer meal. Add your fresh herbs or greens on top of the seeds and drizzle in the olive oil and lemon juice. Pulse again to combine the herbs and pumpkin seeds. Add more oil or lemon juice if needed. The lemon juice will help keep the pesto bright green while also adding a fresh, bright flavor. Use right away or store the pesto in a wide-mouth mason jar, adding a thin layer of extra olive oil on the top before you seal the jar. It will stay fresh for up to 1 week in the fridge. ■

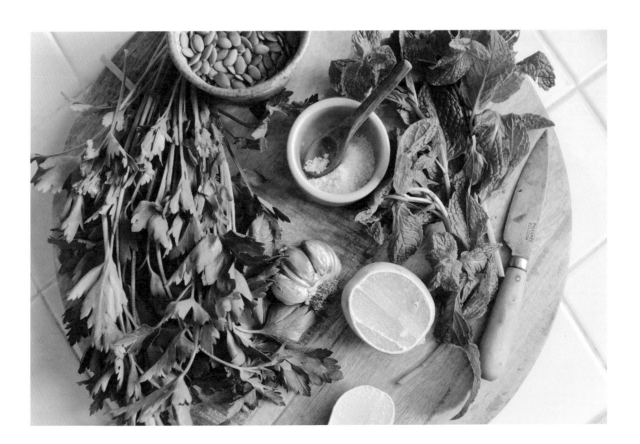

Herbal Vinegars

At the height of summer when our favorite aromatic and mineral-rich herbs are abundant, you'll find us making big batches of herbal vinegars. Freshly dug roots such as burdock and dandelion make delicious vinegars come fall too. Preserving plants in vinegar is an age-old tradition that adds flavor and beneficial microbes to our meals. Apple cider vinegar is our preferred choice, as it can be used in an array of recipes and pairs nicely with most herbs. Herbal vinegars are easy to make and inexpensive while adding a special touch to ordinary dishes. We use them in all kinds of ways: dressings, sauces, a few splashes on rice and beans, bubbly drinks, and even as a hair rinse. FILLS 1 QUART-SIZED JAR

2 to 3 cups fresh and wilted herbs, chopped, or ½ to 1 cup dried herbs

1 quart apple cider vinegar

Fill a quart-sized mason jar with the herbs and pour over the apple cider vinegar. If making a fresh herb vinegar, make sure the vinegar covers the plants by about 1 inch or so, leaving room at the top for expansion. Generally, when using fresh herbs, it's a 2-to-1 ratio, meaning that for every 2 cups of vinegar, you use 1 cup of fresh herbs. Let sit for 1 to 2 weeks in a cool, dry place, giving it a little shake once a day.

Strain through a muslin cloth or mesh strainer and compost or discard the herbs and store the vinegar in a clean jar with a tight-fitting lid. In order to prevent oxidation, cut a square piece of parchment paper to create a barrier between the metal lid and the vinegar, or use a durable and reusable plastic mason jar lid. We store fresh herb vinegars in the fridge for up to 1 month and dried herb vinegars will stay fresh for up to 6 months.

+ SAFETY: It's best to wash, dry, and wilt the fresh herbs a day ahead of time, so they have less water content. The more water, the greater the possibility the vinegar will go bad and grow bacteria. ■

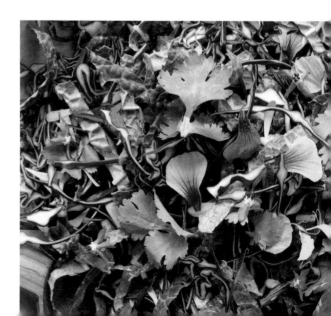

Herbal Dressings

Dressings are more than just for drizzling over salad. They can take stress-soothing and mineral-rich herbs to the next level while giving a comforting grain-and-greens bowl a burst of flavor. Another benefit of herbal dressings is that they involve healthy raw oils that not only bring their own flavor but also aid in supporting healthy hydration and cell, brain, and hormone health. Many of us get enough saturated fat in our diet through animal protein, dairy, or coconut oil. But making sure that we get enough raw oils (especially from seeds) is important to maintain plump, hydrated cells for our skin, hair, and nails, as well as for nervous system health. Here are some of our favorite Kosmic Kitchen staple dressings.

Turmeric Tahini Dressing

FILLS 1 PINT-SIZED JAR

¼ cup apple cider vinegar

Juice of 1 lemon

1½ teaspoons ground turmeric

⅓ cup tahini

Pinch of sea salt

1 cup extra virgin olive, sesame, or sunflower oil

1 garlic clove, minced

½ tablespoon raw local honey or maple syrup

Pour the apple cider vinegar and lemon juice into a small mixing bowl. Whisk in the turmeric, tahini, and salt and continue to whisk vigorously as you slowly pour in the oil. Then mix in the minced garlic and sweetener of choice.

When making a bigger batch of the dressing, it's especially important to slowly pour in the olive oil as you whisk. Slowly adding the oil to the vinegar while whisking is what creates a creamy, emulsified dressing. You can also use a blender to make it super smooth. Add more lemon juice or apple cider vinegar as needed, if it needs more acidity. We store it in the fridge in a mason jar or storage jar with a tight-fitting lid. It will keep for up to 1 week; give it a few shakes before each use. This creamy and dairy-free dressing goes well on warm grain-and-greens bowls; see also our Buckwheat Soba Salad with Turmeric Tahini Dressing (page 162). Simply use more tahini to thicken the dressing and transform it into a dip for roasted veggies. ■

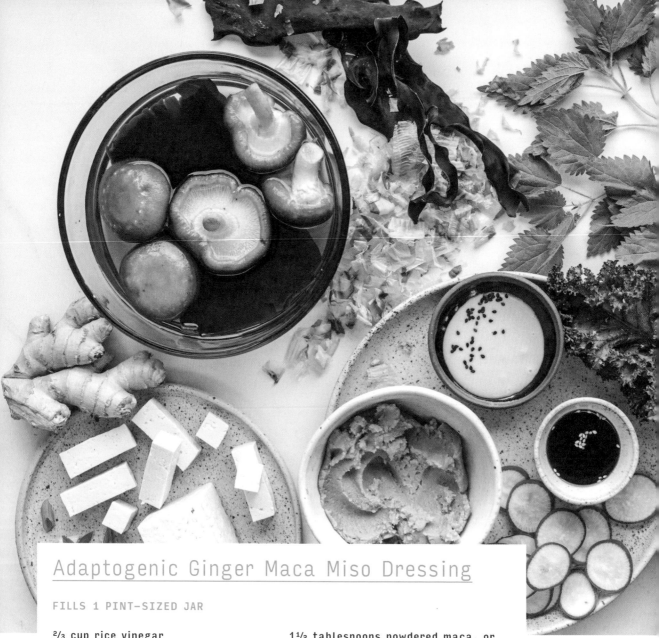

Adaptogenic Ginger Maca Miso Dressing

FILLS 1 PINT-SIZED JAR

²/₃ cup rice vinegar

½ cup olive oil

¼ cup sesame oil

1½ tablespoons white miso

1½ tablespoons powdered maca, or adaptogen of choice

1½-inch thumb fresh ginger, grated

1 tablespoon raw local honey

Add all ingredients to a blender and blend on high speed until combined, or use a hand whisk to blend. To hand whisk, first combine the vinegar and miso. Vigorously whisk in the remaining ingredients, then slowly pour in the oil while continuing to whisk. Store the dressing in a pint-sized mason or storage jar with a tight-fitting lid for up to 1 week; shake a few times before each use. If you

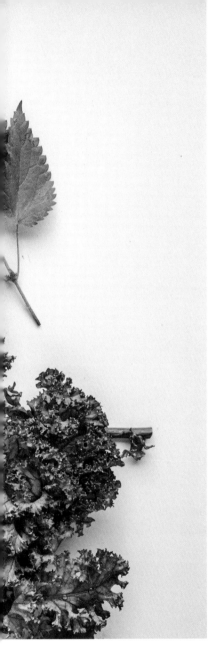

want to thicken the dressing, whisk in a small spoonful or more of miso paste. This tangy ginger dressing goes well with Crispy Salmon with Adaptogenic Ginger Maca Miso Sauce and Roasted Radishes with Herb Butter (page 198), as an alternative dressing for our crunchy Rainbow Salad (page 133), as a flavorful dressing to any salad, or thickened and smeared onto avocado toast with a runny egg.

+ NOTE: Please add in an adaptogen that works best for your dosha. Maca is sweet and nutty, and slightly warming energetically. You may wish to skip the adaptogenic powders altogether or opt for something more cooling such as shatavari. You can always add in fewer powdered herbs, as some of the adaptogens will transform the dressing's taste. ■

Sweet and Sour Ume Plum Dressing

FILLS 1 PINT-SIZED JAR

4 tablespoons umeboshi plum paste

Juice of 3 to 4 limes or lemons

1 to 2 tablespoons raw local honey or maple syrup, to taste

1 cup olive oil

In a small mixing bowl, whisk together the umeboshi plum paste, citrus juice, and sweetener of choice until well combined. Vigorously whisk the mixture while slowly adding in the oil. Taste and adjust by adding more of any of the flavors as desired. Store the dressing in a pint-sized mason or storage jar with a tight-fitting lid for up to 1 week in the fridge; shake a few times before each use. This sour, enzymatic dressing has an addictive umami flavor and goes well with our Rainbow Salad (page 133), in a cooling cucumber salad, or even over grain bowls with roasted veggies or massaged greens. ■

Herbal Honey

Humans have used honey as a sacred food and medicine for thousands of years. This golden nectar, which is food for humans and bees alike, is rich in vitamins, minerals, antioxidants, and enzymes. Egyptians, who observed bees and their hives closely, used honey as a salve and antimicrobial to dress wounds; and they used propolis, a waxy substance bees make and use to seal and protect the hive, to embalm. Ayurvedic texts tell us that honey supports the digestive system. It's commonly used orally to administer medicines and topically to heal cuts and burns. In Chinese medicine, certain herbs are prepared with honey, such as honey-fried astragalus roots, to enhance the tonifying or building energy of the herb. We find that using honey is a delicious way to enjoy medicine, which is why we love to create *melitas*, or medicated honeys. Making medicated honey can be as simple as mixing enzymatic herbs and spices or powdered adaptogens into your honey.

When making herbal honey, look for raw local honey, as it will have the greatest medicinal value because the bees are using the flora where you live. A daily ritual of having 1 teaspoon of raw local honey is said to help the body acclimate to seasonal allergies and stressors. If you have more of a pitta constitution, use honey sparingly, as it's warming in nature. On the other hand, honey (when used in moderation) is great for reducing kapha in the body, which is one reason honey is added to cold and flu teas.

Making a jar of herbal honey every week or so has been a sweet kitchen hack when it comes to making a quick healing tea, adding a hint of sweetness to a dressing, or adding a drizzle over roasted fruit. We typically make each batch in a half-pint-sized mason jar and stir the herbs right in, so there's no mess. Herbal honey is a great way to start experimenting with combining herbs and understanding how their flavors play to their actions in the body. For instance, you'll notice that adjusting the amounts of pungent or bitter versus astringent herbs will create different sensations. From there it's easy to adjust the flavors to your liking. This easy recipe uses spices you probably already have on hand, though you can find more inspiration for your own herbal honey from the list of herbs and spices below.

Turmeric Spice Honey

MAKES ABOUT 1 CUP

½ tablespoon ground turmeric

1 teaspoon ground cardamom

½ teaspoon ground cinnamon

½ teaspoon ground ginger

1 cup raw local honey

In a wide-mouth half-pint-sized mason jar, add in your ground spices and mix to combine. Next, pour in your honey slowly until the jar is about 1 inch from being full. Using a chopstick or the handle of a spoon, stir the herbs and honey until they're well mixed. Add a little more honey once the herbs are combined to fill the jar. Close with a tight-fitting lid and let the honey infuse until ready to use, or enjoy immediately. Use within 3 months. ▪

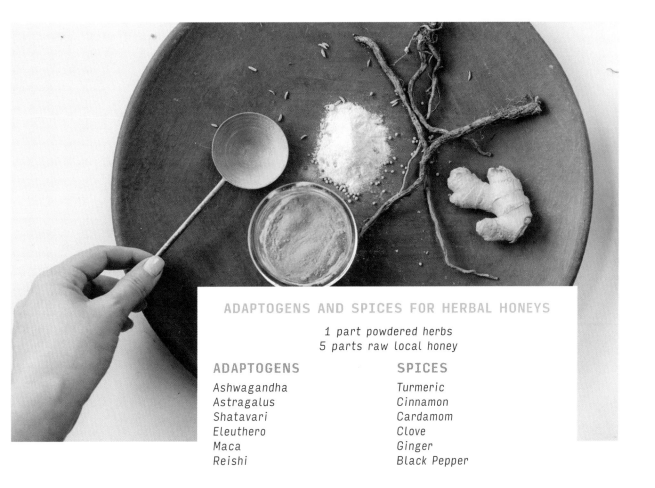

ADAPTOGENS AND SPICES FOR HERBAL HONEYS

1 part powdered herbs
5 parts raw local honey

ADAPTOGENS

Ashwagandha
Astragalus
Shatavari
Eleuthero
Maca
Reishi

SPICES

Turmeric
Cinnamon
Cardamom
Clove
Ginger
Black Pepper

Ghee

Ghee is a sacred medicine in Ayurvedic tradition. For thousands of years, its nourishing properties have worked on the *ojas*, or the subtle essence of all tissues, which is the life force of immunity. The ojas feeds the bone marrow, nerve tissue, brain, subtle tissues of the body, and reproductive tissues. Ghee's magic not only helps our physical body but our mind as well. Dr. Vasant Lad also speaks of ghee giving nourishment to the *tejas*, or the fire of the mind, helping to increase intelligence and perception.

Unsalted butter is transformed into ghee through simple heating, which clarifies the butter by removing hard-to-digest fat solids. Because it's easy to digest (even for many who are lactose intolerant), ghee supports the elemental fire energy of the liver by strengthening it, rather than aggravating it as other oils and fats do. Ghee isn't just an internal medicine; it's also soothing when applied lightly to the skin, eyes, and hair.

Since the energy of ghee is kapha in nature—soothing, building, and grounding—it benefits pitta and vata aggravations. Ghee is calming to the nerves and stimulating for digestive fire, which makes it a wonderful ally for the cold and dry person or during a cold and dry season. FILLS 1 PINT-SIZED JAR

1 pound unsalted organic or local grass-fed butter

Add the butter to a small pot on medium heat. Once it begins to melt, it will look like it's boiling, with a lot of bubbles and foam on the top. Wait about 15 minutes, until the sounds of the boiling change and the appearance of the bubbles gets smaller and more dispersed. Gently push away a section of bubbles with a wooden spoon to peek at the milk solids that have fallen to the bottom to make sure they aren't burning. Remove from the heat and let the ghee cool for a few minutes, then skim off the foam at the top with a spoon into a pint-sized jar. Strain the ghee into the jar with cheesecloth or a mesh strainer to prevent the milk solids from getting into the now clarified butter. Seal the jar with a tight lid and let cool completely.

Keep your ghee on the counter or in the pantry so it's easy to spoon out for daily use. There's no need to store it in the fridge, as it's shelf stable. Make sure to only use clean utensils when scooping it from the jar to prevent moisture from spoiling the ghee. ∎

Herbal Ghee

Herbal powders can also be infused in ghee. In this preparation, ghee is like a vehicle for herbs to penetrate body tissues because of its nutritive and building qualities. The traditional way of making herbal ghee involves a water decoction method, but it can be difficult to ensure all the water is removed, which can lead to rancid ghee. To avoid the ghee going bad and to save time, you can infuse powdered herbs with the butter while it's clarifying.

We tend to stick to adaptogenic powders for their building qualities and affinity with the nervous system. Infuse 1 ounce of adaptogen powder (a mix or just one) with 1 pound of unsalted butter by placing the butter in saucepan and sprinkling the herbs on top. From here, you can follow the steps for making plain ghee, including straining and storage, on page 110.

Healing Broths

Broths are foundational to our kosmic kitchen, and we love compounding their benefits by adding in adaptogens, mushrooms, and seaweeds. We often use these broths in which to cook our grains and porridge, and as a base for our soups and stews. They can also be sipped like tea in the heart of winter. These broths can be made ahead in bulk and stored in the freezer for later use, that way you have them handy when you need them in a pinch.

Everyday Herbal Bone Broth

FILLS 3 TO 4 QUART-SIZED JARS

2 pounds of chicken bones, include chicken feet for extra gelatin

3 celery stalks, chopped

3 carrots, chopped

3 cloves garlic, smashed

3 bay leaves

1 onion, chopped

2 tablespoons apple cider vinegar

1 handful fresh rosemary and/or thyme

4 slices astragalus root, optional

3-inch thumb fresh ginger, chopped

Sea salt, optional

Add all the ingredients and about 1 gallon of water into a large pot. Cover and bring to a boil, then reduce heat to allow the mixture to simmer on low for 3 to 4 hours; you can also use a slow cooker for this. If you have the time and would like to do a longer broth that slow-cooks for 6 to 8 hours, hold off on adding the veggies and herbs until the last 3 to 4 hours of cooking. You can tell the broth is done once it's rich and flavorful. Then strain out the veggies, spices, and bones. Allow the broth to cool before pouring into glass jars for storing, or else you risk breaking the glass. Store in the fridge if you plan to use within the next few days. The broth will become thick and gelatinous when cold, which is the sign of a super nourishing bone broth that's filled with gut-healing gelatin. If not using immediately, store in the freezer for up to 3 months.

+ NOTE: When using this recipe for stock, it's best to skip the salt; that way you can have more wiggle room for flavor when using it as a base for a soup recipe. ▪

Mineral-Rich Seaweed and Mushroom Broth

FILLS 3 TO 4 QUART-SIZED JARS

3 carrots, chopped

3 celery stalks, chopped

3 cloves garlic, smashed

3 sweet potatoes, chopped

1 leek, chopped

2 bay leaves

Three 8-inch slices kombu

1 onion, chopped

6 ounces fresh shiitake mushrooms, chopped

½ bunch parsley, chopped

½ bunch fresh nettle or wild green of choice, when in season

½ tablespoon whole peppercorns

1 gallon water

Add all the ingredients into a large pot. Cover the pot and bring to a boil, then reduce the heat and allow the mixture to simmer on low for 2 to 3 hours; you can also use a slow cooker for this. Once the broth tastes rich, it's done cooking. Then, strain out the veggies, spices, mushrooms, and seaweed. Allow the broth to cool before pouring into glass jars for storing, or else you risk breaking the glass. Store in the fridge if you plan to use within the next few days or keep it in the freezer for up to 3 months.

+ NOTE: When using this recipe for stock, it's best to skip the salt; that way you can have more wiggle room for flavor when using it as a base for a soup recipe. Plus, this seaweed-infused broth is naturally salty on its own.

Herbal Power Bites

We were first introduced to these easy-to-make medicine bites by the esteemed herbalist Rosemary Gladstar, who traditionally uses stimulating herbs to make what she calls "zoom balls." Rosemary is all about finding delicious ways to eat your medicine every day, and as our teacher, she has deeply influenced our kitchen herbalism practice. These little bites are filled not only with medicinal herbs but also greens powder—like the kind you'd normally toss into a smoothie—that is packed with mineral- and vitamin-rich plants. We call them "herbal powder bites" because these herbs are mostly restorative and building, giving us steady power through the week.

We're more called to savory snacks than sweet ones, and these bites are packed with much more flavor than just the sweetness of honey. Once you make a batch for the week, you can blend a few with your favorite smoothie, spread them on warm toast for a quick breakfast, or pack a few in your bag for a snack. Each ingredient has a benefit. Sunflower butter provides not only plant protein but also lecithin, a fat essential to nourishing the myelin sheath that covers nerve endings and supports the nervous system. The greens powder is a combination of superfoods and herbs high in vitamins, trace minerals, chlorophyll, antioxidants, and enzymes.

When making this recipe, think about the energetics you need to balance and which herbs or flavors would support the opposite quality. This is another great way to experiment with simple formulations based around the herbs and spices with which you're building a relationship. For instance, if you're noticing more symptoms of cold and dry, add moistening and warming herbs such as ashwagandha, cinnamon, and ginger. If it's summer or if you have a pitta constitution, lean on cooling and bitter herbs such as turmeric, fennel, and shatavari root as part of your herbal blend. MAKES 25 BITES, AND EACH SERVING HAS ABOUT A SINGLE DOSE OF ADAPTOGENS

2 cups sunflower butter, or seed or nut butter of choice

¾ cup raw local honey

⅓ cup adaptogenic powder(s) of choice

2 tablespoons greens powder (we like Healthforce Vitamineral Green)

1 teaspoon ground cardamom

1 teaspoon ground cinnamon

1 teaspoon ground ginger

Pinch of sea salt

Toasted coconut flakes, optional

Cacao powder, optional

Ground cayenne, optional

In a mixing bowl, add all the ingredients and combine into a paste. The texture should feel a bit like cookie dough. If it feels too dry, simply add a little more honey to moisten. With your hands, roll the dough into bite-sized balls, about 1 inch in diameter, and place them in a container with parchment paper between each layer to prevent them from sticking together. To prevent sticky hands, you may wish to wet your hands before rolling out the balls.

You can leave them plain, or coat with a little toasted coconut or raw cacao powder, if you'd like. Sprinkle with a touch of cayenne for extra spice. Store in a container with a tight-fitting lid. They will keep for about 1 week in the fridge or about 1 month in the freezer. ■

Miso Immune Soup Balls

Much like our Herbal Power Bites recipe (page 114), these soup balls are quick and easy. You can make them ahead of time, then simply heat them up in a simmering pot of water and add in whatever extra goodness you like. Try them in our Miso Immune Soup with Astragalus, Burdock, and Shiitake (page 229) for an example of how you might use them in a meal. **MAKES ABOUT 12 BALLS**

¼ cup dried wakame seaweed

¼ cup black sesame seeds

2 cups miso paste, we like barley miso for cooler months

2 tablespoons astragalus powder

3-inch thumb fresh ginger, grated

Put the seaweed and sesame seeds into a food processor or coffee grinder. Pulse until roughly ground, or grind them more finely if you'd like. In a large mixing bowl, and using a wooden spoon or spatula, combine the mixture with the miso, astragalus powder, and ginger. Using the palms of your hands, ideally wet to prevent sticking, roll the paste into 2-inch balls and place in an airtight container with parchment paper to separate the layers. You will use these almost like bouillon cubes. Store in the freezer for up to 3 months. ■

PART

3

"Is there any practice less selfish, any labor less alienated, any time less wasted, than preparing something delicious and nourishing for people you love?"

—MICHAEL POLLAN

RECIPES FOR RADICAL WELLNESS

NOW THAT YOU HAVE A SENSE OF HOW A KOSMIC KITCHEN comes together, let's explore some of our favorite recipes throughout the seasons. The next section of recipes is intended for you to flip through and find inspiration during any time of year. Each season also serves as a reminder as to which elements will be in excess and the need to balance with the opposite energy. We encourage you to see the recipes as starting points, using what you already have in your kitchen and pantry, but also to feel confident trying new flavors in different ways. Makes these recipes your own. Get creative and put your own unique spin on which herbs and ingredients you use, based on what's growing in your garden or fresh from your bioregion.

When we're in the kitchen, cooking becomes a way to connect with our senses and intuition. On a deeper level, cooking is about strengthening the connection you have to your body and internal knowing. This is what we call radical wellness—being able to listen and trust your internal knowing to guide you toward what feels the most healing to you. It's easy to get swept up in the latest wellness fad, but when you're grounded in yourself and honor the messages your body tells you, you'll be amazed at how nourishing the simplest remedies can feel and how effective they can be.

You'll also notice we give self-care rituals for each season to create holistic everyday practices, both internally and externally. Taking time to connect with your body each day, whether you have three hours for a full-on self-care routine or fifteen minutes to do a quick self-oil massage, is an important pillar of feeling well. See these rituals as inspiration to create your own favorite practices that feel and work best for you.

SPRING

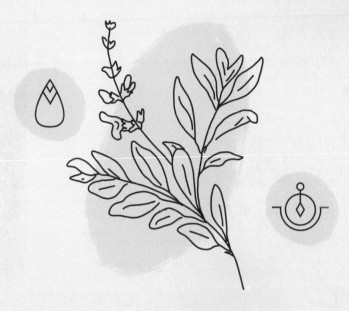

JUST WHEN IT FEELS AS THOUGH YOU CAN BARELY STAND another cold, gray day, little blades of green begin to pop up as reminders that warmer, brighter days are near. Spring can be a wonderful season of renewal and growth. All winter long we've been nestled quietly in the darkness, dreaming, so we can have the clarity to plant the seeds in our lives and watch them grow.

In every season, nature provides us with cues to align our bodies with the environment around us. Enjoying foods that are lighter, warming, and stimulating—as opposed to heavy, building foods from the winter season—will give our bodies support to transition into spring with ease. Light, mineral-rich soups, bitter greens with drying and cleansing properties, and spices all help stimulate our immune and digestive systems to function optimally, and they also help our bodies release any excess fluid or heaviness we've accumulated during the cold, wet winter months. This is a time to let go of any foods that are no longer serving us, giving our bodies a break to naturally cleanse as we head into the warmer months. It's also a wonderful time to start incorporating more fresh foods as they become more abundant.

Creating weekly rituals that are stimulating, invigorating, and nourishing to our bodies will help us not just release physical stagnation but also create space for new possibilities. This is the time to stretch, move, and open from the dark womb of winter, blossoming into spring and the abundance this season brings.

FOODS	HERBS	RITUALS	REDUCE
Light, stimulating, and warming cooked foods, such as miso soups and porridges, with a mix of fresh and steamed veggies	Aromatic and warming spices: cayenne, cinnamon, garlic, ginger, rosemary, sage, thyme, turmeric	Warming Winter Salt Scrub (page 244)	Sweet and salty foods
		Warm baths to relax and promote circulation	Wet, heavy, and dense foods, or things that are high in saturated fats
Lots of spices to support the circulatory system in staying warm	Cleansing and lymphatic system herbs: burdock, chickweed, cleavers, dandelion greens, red clover	Dry Brushing (page 145) to support the lymphatic system	Cow dairy products
		Walk outside after meals	Eating heavy meals and snacking throughout the day
Raw fresh fruits and fiber-rich veggies to stimulate the digestive system and support systems of elimination	Warming adaptogens: ashwagandha, maca, eleuthero, schisandra, tulsi	Cardio to break a sweat and move the lymph	Eating as a way of coping emotionally
		Breath work to stay embodied	Overextending yourself

SPRING SEASON

ELEMENTS: Water and Earth

QUALITIES: Cold and Wet

DOSHA: Kapha

BALANCING FLAVORS: Astringent, bitter, pungent, sour

SIGNS OF BALANCE: Feeling energized and grounded, open to new possibilities, staying warm and having good circulation

SIGNS OF IMBALANCE: Feeling cold, damp, heavy, depressed, sensitive; having excess fluids and mucus, runny nose, sluggish digestion with low digestive fire

Everyday Spring Brew

Teas are a great way to create an everyday herbal practice that provides healing and connects you with the plants. Rosemary Gladstar, once told us, "If you don't have time to make yourself tea, I can't help you." In her loving and direct way, she is saying that if you can't find the time to pause, take your medicines, and practice self-love, you may not get the results you're looking for.

For many, an everyday herbal tea ritual sounds too simple to be effective. But these subtle herbal medicines accumulate over time. That's why we like to make a big batch of a healing blend, so we have it handy throughout the season.

This tea features a nourishing blend of roots, leaves, and flowers. It's a restorative, with a heavy dose of nettle to promote kidney, liver, and digestive system health. Because nettle leaf supports the systems of elimination and the bitter dandelion root activates the digestive enzymes, this blend is perfect to enjoy after a sluggish winter season. The lightly demulcent calendula flowers support and hydrate the mucous membranes of the digestive system, and the astringency of the rose petals tone and tighten tissue—and add some energetic heart healing to the blend. FILLS 1 PINT-SIZED JAR

$2/3$ **cup nettle leaf, dried**

$1/3$ **cup calendula petals, dried**

6 tablespoons rose petals, dried

2 tablespoons dandelion root, dried

2 teaspoons cinnamon bark or ginger, dried for flavor; optional

2 teaspoons licorice, dried; optional (see safety note)

+ SAFETY: **Please avoid licorice if you have high blood pressure. If you still desire sweetness, add a bit of honey, to taste.**

+ NOTE: **All herbs and flowers should be cut and sifted.**

Add herbs to a bowl or jar and mix well with a spoon. Store in a jar with a tight-fitting lid to keep the herbs fresh for use over the next couple weeks. Create a label for the jar with details on the date made and what herbs were used.

To make a daily quart of tea, add 2 to 3 tablespoons (about 1 teaspoon or more per cup) of the blend to a muslin bag or tea pouch of choice and then place inside a quart-sized mason jar. Preheat the jar with warm water on the outside, then fill with hot water for tea. Cover and allow the mixture to infuse for 15 to 20 minutes or so; use the Hot Water Herbal Infusion recipe (page 94) as inspiration. Remove the muslin bag or tea pouch, add honey or lemon to taste, if desired, and enjoy this spring tea throughout the day. We suggest sipping on about 2 to 4 cups throughout the day to get the most benefit. Store in the fridge for up to 2 days. ■

Tulsi Matcha Latte

On cool spring mornings, there's nothing like the flavor of creamy pumpkin milk to accompany the bright flavors of tulsi and matcha. Tulsi is one of our favorite herbs to enjoy as a simple tea, but it's also excellent in pesto, dressings, or added freshly chopped to top a meal. By blending this herb with matcha, the ceremonial Japanese powdered green tea that's recently exploded in popularity, you'll be able to enjoy the grounded calm that tulsi provides along with the stimulating benefits of the matcha for alertness and energy. MAKES 1 CUP

½ cup tulsi tea; see Hot Water Herbal Infusions (page 94)

¼ teaspoon matcha powder

½ cup pumpkin seed milk or milk of choice; see "What to Do with

Soaked and Sprouted Nuts and Seeds" (page 90)

1 teaspoon raw local honey or sweetener of choice

Warm the tulsi tea in a small saucepan; you want it to be hot but not boiling. Add the matcha powder to a mug, then slowly pour in a small splash of the warm tulsi tea. Using a bamboo whisk, mix the matcha powder and tea until the matcha is smooth, forming a thin paste and making sure there aren't any clumps. Add in the rest of the tulsi tea and continue to whisk until well blended. Warm your milk in the same small pot and add your sweetener, then pour the mixture into the tulsi matcha. Enjoy warm in the morning or in the afternoon for a soothing pick-me-up. ▪

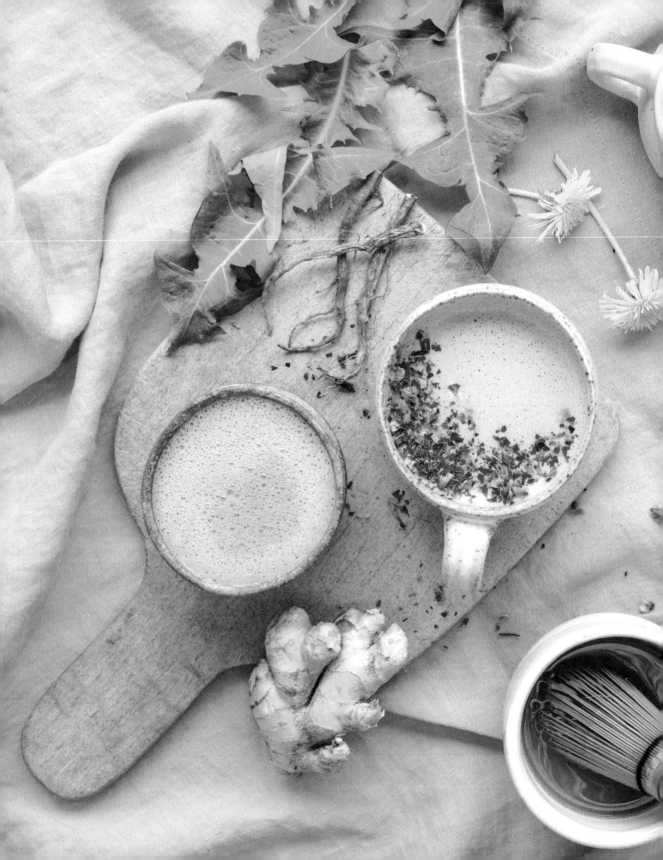

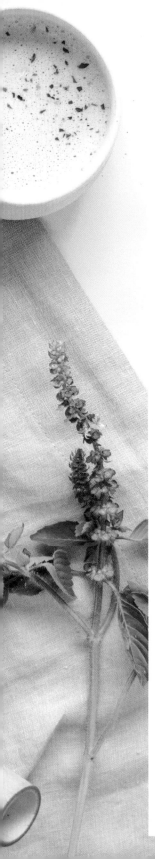

Roasted Dandelion Chai Concentrate

If you're looking for a morning pick-me-up without the caffeine, try this sweet and spicy chai with roasted dandelion root. Dandelion is a traditional spring tonic and bitter herb that supports the liver and the digestive system. By supporting our systems of elimination, dandelion helps our bodies get rid of what we don't need and allows for rejuvenation and gentle cleansing. FILLS 1 QUART-SIZED JAR

6 cups water

3½ tablespoons cut and sifted, dried roasted dandelion root

2 cinnamon sticks

2-inch thumb fresh ginger, sliced

1 teaspoon whole cloves

1 tablespoon cardamom pods

3 whole star anise

2 teaspoons vanilla extract

3 to 4 tablespoons raw local honey, or another sweetener of choice to taste

Plant milk of your choice, warmed and frothed; optional (see below)

Pour the water into a large pot with a lid, bring to a boil, and then reduce down to a simmer. Add in all the ingredients except the vanilla extract, honey, and plant milk. Cover and allow the mixture to decoct (see page 96) for 20 to 30 minutes. Turn off the burner and allow the chai to cool a bit. Strain out the herbs using a mesh strainer or French press, add the vanilla extract and honey, and store in a quart-sized mason jar to enjoy over the next few days. You can serve the beverage hot or cold with the plant milk of your choice at a 1-to-1 ratio. This mixture will stay fresh in the fridge for up to 3 days.

Latte Milk

To make a milky froth, we like to use a blender or a frother. You can create a nut or seed milk from scratch; see our recipe at "What to Do with Soaked and Sprouted Nuts and Seeds" (page 90). Add whatever milk you choose to your blender and blend for about 1 minute; this will create a frothy latte-like consistency. If you're a latte lover, we suggest investing in a Breville frother, or simply use an inexpensive hand frother to create your frothed milk separately to then add to your hot latte. ■

Rose Cinnamon Tahini Milk

This simple, warming, and floral seed milk is a life changer. For anyone who doesn't have the patience to make nut milks, this recipe is for you. Tahini, or sesame seed paste, is another staple in our kitchens, though it's mostly used in savory dishes, dips, and dressings. Here, the nutty and slightly bitter tahini is transformed into a delicious drink with the help of cinnamon and rose. Enjoy a cup on its own or blend with your favorite powdered adaptogens to make a truly decadent healing beverage. FILLS 1 QUART-SIZED JAR

¼ cup raw tahini

1 tablespoon dried organic rose petals or 1 teaspoon rose water

2 dates, pitted

½ teaspoon ground cinnamon

¼ teaspoon sea salt, or more, to taste

4 cups water

Add all the ingredients to a high-speed blender and blend on high for 1 to 2 minutes. Taste and adjust the flavor to your liking, if needed. Add more sea salt a pinch at a time until it brings out the nuttiness of the tahini and sweetness from the dates. Store the milk in a quart-sized mason jar in the fridge, if not using immediately. The milk will stay fresh in the fridge for up to 4 days. Shake well before using, as separation can occur. ▪

Overnight Oats: Sweet and Savory

We love soaking our oats overnight to make them easier to digest and more bioavailable. The process also gives the porridge a creamier consistency and an interesting tangy twist. Most of us have grown up with the classic bowl of oats accompanied by dried fruit, nuts, and sugar. We encourage you to try something different. Incorporate adaptogenic powders for your constitution, cook the oats in broth, and incorporate medicinal herbs that feel energetically aligned with the season. SERVES 2

1 cup rolled oats

Water, filtered or unchlorinated preferred (see note)

Salt, to taste

+ NOTE: We suggest using filtered or unchlorinated water and soaking your grains overnight. But please know that any amount of soak time is better than none at all! With this oatmeal recipe, we often use the soaking water to cook the oats, as it adds more flavor.

First, soak your oatmeal in a bowl, covered, overnight. Use 1 part oatmeal to 2 parts water for a thick oatmeal, or 1 part oatmeal to 3 parts water for a creamier, porridge-like consistency. Once the mixture is done soaking, add the oats and soaking water in to a saucepan and bring to a boil. Add salt to taste, and then reduce the heat to a low simmer until the water is absorbed. The cooking time will be reduced drastically due to the soaking process. Make sure to stir the oats occasionally to prevent them from overcooking and sticking to the bottom of the pan. Once finished cooking, the oats will reach a porridge-like consistency.

Your oatmeal will taste a bit acidic, as it has been lightly fermented during the soaking process, so don't be alarmed. You can add sweetener to mellow the flavor. By doing this quick ferment, the oats will be easier to digest and for your body to absorb. See next page for topping suggestions. ■

Recipe photo on following page.

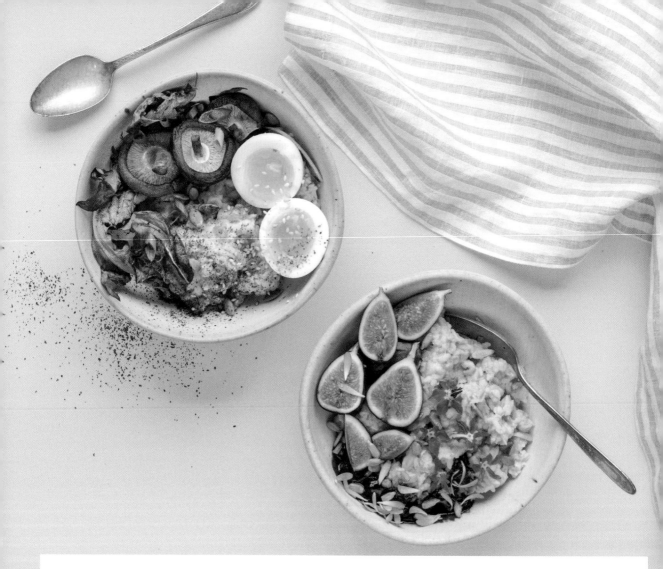

TOPPINGS FOR SWEET

Seasonal spring fruits, including cherries, strawberries, and dried fruits

Herbal honey, maple syrup, or sweetener of choice

Building adaptogens, such as shatavari and maca powder (1 teaspoon per serving)

Digestive supportive spices, such as cinnamon and cardamom

Edible flowers for garnish, such as borage and calendula

TOPPINGS FOR SAVORY

Seasonal steamed or sautéed greens, such as mustard, dandelion, and nettles

Grounding proteins, such as hard-boiled egg or diced tofu

Stimulating and warming spices, such as ginger, turmeric, cayenne, and black pepper

Warming adaptogens, such as ashwagandha, or building adaptogens such as maca powder (1 teaspoon per serving)

Fresh herbs, such as cilantro and green onions

Sea salts, ground seaweed, and tamari or soy sauce for extra flavor

Ginger–Garlic Braised Dandelion Greens

Most days, you will likely find us braising some sort of leafy green to accompany a meal. Whether it's lacinato kale, radicchio, or collards, there's something about the bitter bite of these greens that hits the spot in savory dishes. The bitter flavor stimulates the digestive system, helps release digestive enzymes, and cleanses and supports the liver. If we indulge in too many sweets or fried or fatty foods over the winter months, the liver can work overtime and needs extra support from bitter flavors. Dandelion greens are one of our favorite spring greens, though they can be quite bitter. While bitter is cooling, it can also be cleansing, and this is great to help our bodies slough off excess fluids or heaviness after coming through the dormancy of winter. If you're just introducing more bitter foods to your plate, mix dandelion greens with other dark leafy greens you already enjoy. Using warming herbs known for their antimicrobial and expectorant properties, such as ginger and garlic, is helpful if you're dealing with a cold or flu and need support moving phlegm out of the body. SERVES 2 TO 4

2 teaspoons Ghee (page 110) or coconut oil

1 garlic clove, finely minced

1 bunch dandelion greens, kale or collards, rinsed and roughly chopped

1 tablespoon tamari

1 teaspoon maple syrup

1-inch thumb fresh ginger, grated

½ tablespoon toasted sesame oil

Sprinkle of flake salt, to taste

In a cast-iron skillet, heat the ghee on medium-low until melted. Add garlic and cook for about 1 minute, just until softened and fragrant but not browned. Add the dandelion greens, tossing them with the ghee and garlic until they're bright green and wilted. Turn off the heat.

In a small bowl, combine the tamari, maple syrup, ginger, and toasted sesame oil and whisk together. Pour the sauce over the dandelion greens, coating them thoroughly. With a pair of tongs, add the greens to a plate, pour the remaining sauce in the pan over the top, and sprinkle on the flake salt. Enjoy these as a side dish, in a grain bowl, or on sourdough toast with eggs for breakfast. ■

Kitchari with Golden Ghee

Kitchari is an ancient dish of rice and mung dahl or lentils with spices. In Ayurvedic medicine, kitchari is seen as a healing food during *panchakarma*, the cleansing and rejuvenating program for the mind, body, and consciousness. Kitchari is given to patients throughout this weeklong program because it's high in protein, vitamins, and complex carbohydrates, and it's easily digested. While spring is considered an ideal time to cleanse postwinter, a panchakarma program can be done at any time to restore balance.

This comforting dish has been a mainstay in our kitchen for years. Our version is adapted from *The Yoga of Herbs* by Dr. David Frawley and Dr. Vasant Lad. Not only is it delicious, filling without being heavy, and quite simple to make, but also each of its spices impart carminative healing benefits. Carminatives support healthy digestion and peristalsis while helping to relieve gas and intestinal pain. SERVES 4

2 tablespoons Ghee (page 110) or coconut oil

2 teaspoons mustard seeds

2 teaspoons fennel seeds

2 teaspoons ground coriander

2 teaspoons ground cumin

2 teaspoons ground turmeric

1 cup basmati rice, soaked overnight and rinsed (see page 88)

2 cups mung beans, soaked overnight and rinsed (see page 88)

6 cups water

In a large stock pot, melt the ghee over medium heat, then add the mustard and fennel seeds and sauté until they begin to pop. Add the coriander, cumin, and turmeric, along with the rice and mung beans, and stir until coated. Next, pour in water and give a good stir, bring to a simmer, and cook, covered, for 20 to 30 minutes, or until rice is cooked and mung beans are soft. ■

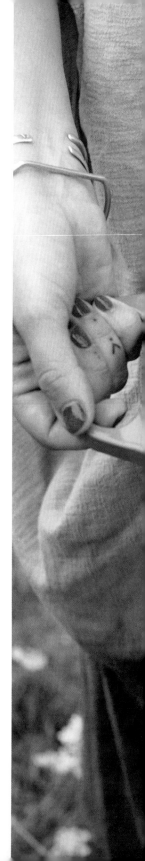

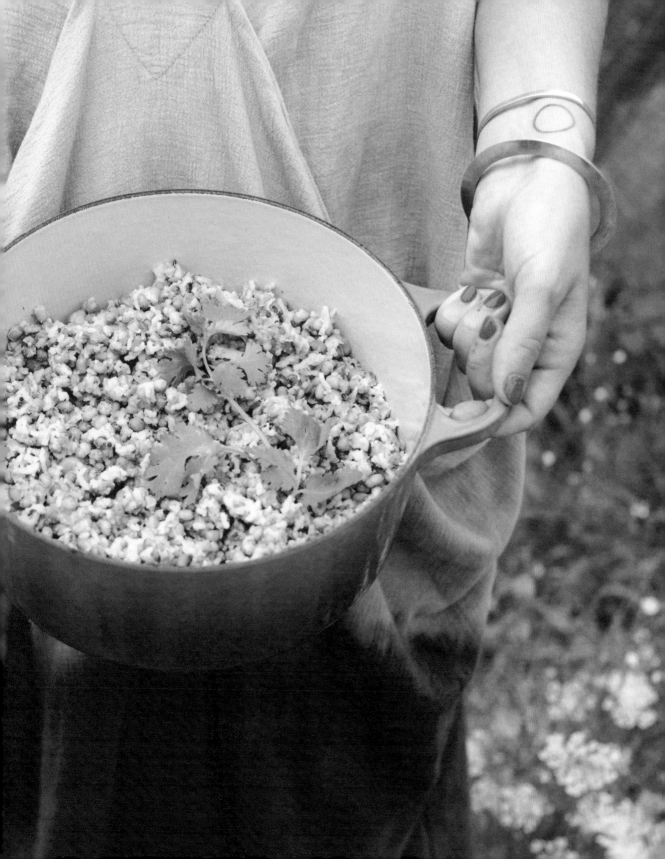

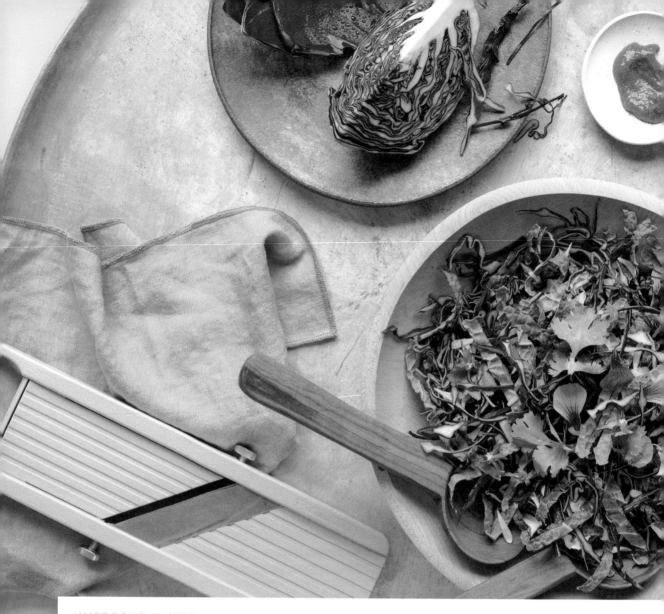

UMEBOSHI PLUMS

Said to be the Japanese equivalent of "an apple a day," umeboshi plums are a popular staple that is infused in everything from vinegars to pastes. Umeboshi plum paste can be found throughout Japan and in most health food stores here in the United States, somewhat due to the popular macrobiotic diet. Ume means "plum," but the fruit, which is in the Rosaceae family, is actually more closely related to the apricot. The fruits are picked in late spring while still green, sour, and unripe.

The key to ume preservation occurs through a salt ferment. The relationship between the citric acid in the fruit combined with sea salt creates a highly enzymatic fermented food and medicine that supports the liver and aids in digestion. In traditional foods, this medicinal paste is used like a condiment, in pastes and vinegars, and served on everything from salads to congee. Ume is seen as both a cold and hangover remedy, infused into teas and liquor drinks, and is revered as a culinary staple worldwide due to its unexpected and delicious salty-sour flavor.

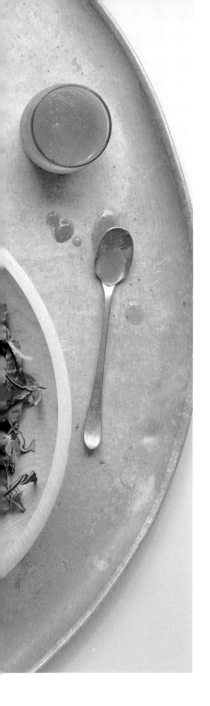

Rainbow Salad with Sweet and Sour Ume Plum Dressing

If you're not familiar with umeboshi plum paste (see opposite), get ready to fall in love. Its sharp, salty, sour, and sweet flavor combination adds the perfect twist to an otherwise simple dressing. Umeboshi plums are a traditional Japanese salt ferment often mixed with purple shiso leaves (*Perilla frutescens*), which is what gives the paste its light-pink hue. The finished ferment, high in vitamin C, is alkalizing, aids fatigue, and helps improve digestion and liver function. This sweet and sour dressing complements the fresh and crunchy cabbage salad and is delightful on its own or with soup on a sunny spring day. SERVES 4

½ **head green or red cabbage**

1 **bunch kale**

1 **bunch cilantro, de-stemmed and whole**

½ **cup dried currants**

½ **cup toasted pumpkin seeds, sunflower seeds, or cashews**

Sweet and Sour Ume Plum Dressing (page 107)

Edible flowers, such as borage, calendula, and nasturtium (page 70)

Using a sharp knife or mandolin, shred the cabbage as thinly as possible into a large salad bowl. De-stem the kale, thinly slice into strips, and add to the bowl. If you prefer to skip kale, add in the rest of the cabbage or buy both red and green to get a rainbowlike look.

   Then add in the whole cilantro leaves, dried currants, and toasted seeds, reserving a handful of each for garnish along with edible flowers. Pour the dressing over the salad, to taste, and toss, making sure everything is well coated. Serve immediately as a solo salad or as part of a bigger lunch spread. If you're making this ahead of time, wait to dress and garnish the salad until serving. ■

Nourishing Nettle Soup with White Beans and Shiitakes

When it's cold and rainy for days on end, nothing is more comforting than a bowl of hot soup. This recipe is packed with some of our favorite nourishing foods and features a delicious spring green—stinging nettle. Usually during this time of year, our bodies need extra support to ward off colds and flus. Soups are a hydrating and warming vehicle, making it easy for herbs to help boost our immune systems and aid in proper elimination of toxins. With a few key ingredients, you can transform a simple soup into a medicinal meal.

Nettle (see page 66) is a wonderful daily tonic with a delicious green flavor perfect to add to a soup. You can find fresh nettle at farmers markets or try your hand at growing it in the garden. For those new to stinging nettle, it's important to handle with care and use gloves. Once cooked, nettle will lose its powerful sting. If you can't track down fresh nettle, substitute hearty greens such as kale or collards. Another mineral-rich food that is easily assimilated, kombu (*Saccharina japonica*) is deeply nourishing while also aiding digestion of proteins and oils. Shiitake mushrooms (*Lentinula edodes*) add a meaty texture to this soup, along with additional immune support. SERVES 4

1 tablespoon Ghee (page 110) or coconut oil

1 sweet onion, diced

2 garlic cloves, smashed and minced

3-inch thumb fresh ginger, grated

2 cups fresh shiitake mushrooms, sliced with stems removed

4 cups cannellini beans, cooked

8-inch strip dried kombu

2 bay leaves

2 quarts Everyday Herbal Bone Broth (page 112) or vegetable broth

4 cups fresh nettle, roughly chopped, stems removed

1 tablespoon chopped fresh thyme

1 tablespoon chopped fresh parsley

Sea salt and freshly cracked black pepper

Olive oil

In a heavy-bottomed pot, melt the ghee, then add the onions and cook until tender. Toss in the garlic, ginger, and shiitakes, stirring until they have a little color and are fragrant. Add in the cannellini beans, kombu, bay leaves, and broth, making sure the ingredients are fully covered by the broth. Stir to

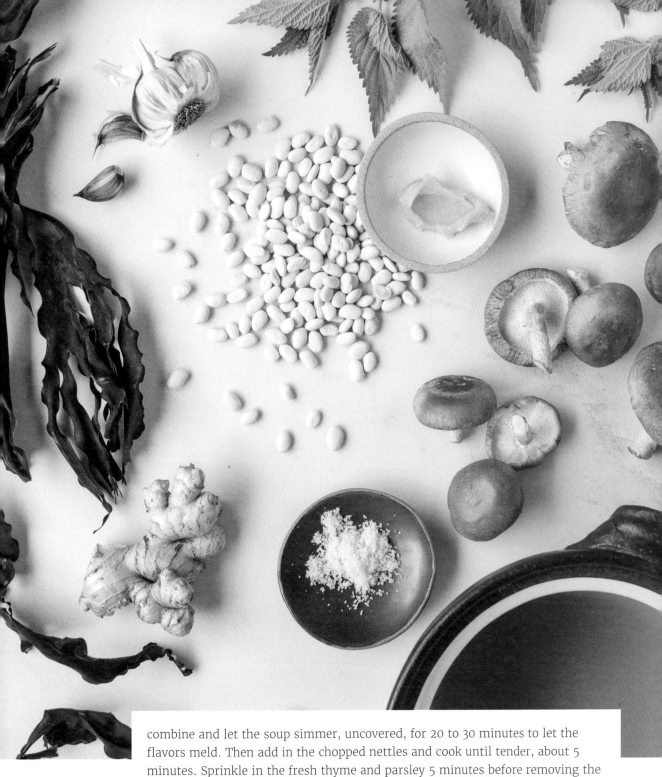

combine and let the soup simmer, uncovered, for 20 to 30 minutes to let the flavors meld. Then add in the chopped nettles and cook until tender, about 5 minutes. Sprinkle in the fresh thyme and parsley 5 minutes before removing the soup from the heat. Ladle into bowls and add salt, pepper, and a drizzle of olive oil for garnish. ■

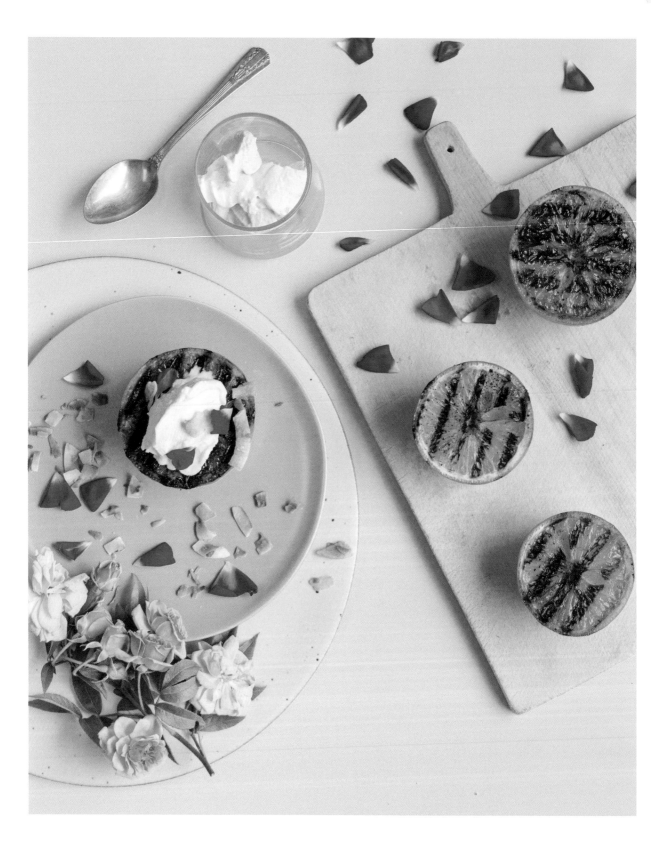

Grilled Oranges with Rose Coconut Cream

Just on the cusp of late winter and early spring, there's an abundance of citrus in California. From blood oranges and Cara Cara oranges to Oro Blanco grapefruit, the flavor of tart-sweet juicy citrus feels like a burst of sunshine during the gray drizzly days. Grilling fruit, especially citrus, brings out a deeper, more complex sweetness and makes for a quick warming dessert. Instead of firing up the outdoor grill, we used a grill pan on the stovetop, so this recipe comes together pretty easily and with little mess. To make this recipe a little more special, we added a rose coconut cream and turmeric coconut crunchies. These golden coconut flakes add an extra pop of color and flavor to this dish. Make a batch to last you for the week to sprinkle on granola and yogurt, a breakfast bowl, or a weeknight curry. SERVES 4

FOR THE TURMERIC COCONUT CRUNCHIES

2 cups coconut flakes, we like the large flakes rather than shredded

1 teaspoon ground turmeric

FOR THE ROSE COCONUT CREAM

One 13.5-ounce can full-fat coconut milk, chilled

1 teaspoon raw local honey

½ tablespoon rose water

FOR THE GRILLED ORANGES

½ tablespoon coconut oil, melted

2 oranges, cut in half down the middle with seeds removed

Drizzle of raw local honey, for garnish

1 tablespoon dried rose petals, crushed, for garnish

For the turmeric coconut crunchies, preheat the oven to 350°F. In a mixing bowl, toss together the coconut flakes and turmeric powder until evenly coated. Spread coconut flakes in an even layer onto a baking sheet lined with parchment paper. Bake until fragrant and toasted, 5 to 7 minutes. Store in a glass jar to keep them fresh.

recipe continues on following page

You can make the rose coconut cream just before grilling the oranges. Simply remove the coconut milk from the fridge and scoop off the top layer of cream, about 1 cup, and add to a bowl or stand mixer. Reserve the rest of the coconut milk to use in another dish. Drizzle in the honey and rose water, and whip with a whisk or in the mixer until combined. Adjust sweetness if needed by adding more honey. Keep in the fridge until ready to serve.

To grill the oranges, brush each cut side with coconut oil and place on a hot grill pan. They only need 1 to 2 minutes for the juice to caramelize and get a little charred. Remove from the grill pan and let cool for a few minutes. Score the oranges around the edges between the pith and the flesh. Cut the flesh into bite-sized sections to make them easier to eat. Serve with a dollop of rose coconut cream and a drizzle of honey, and sprinkle with dried rose petals and turmeric coconut crunchies. ▪

Adaptogenic Ghee– Stuffed Dates

This is our ultimate sweet treat to enjoy without worrying about getting a sugar hangover. The combination of the dried dates with the ghee tastes like rich caramel. Infusing ghee with herbs is an Ayurvedic practice that helps drive the herbs into the tissues of the body. These little stuffed dates make a satisfying snack that comes together with little effort. Double the recipe to make a batch that will last you throughout the week. MAKES 10 STUFFED DATES

10 medjool dates

¼ cup Ghee (page 110), softened at room temperature

2 tablespoons adaptogen powder of choice such as ashwagandha, maca, or shatavari

Pinch of ground cardamom, cinnamon, or ginger

Fresh orange or lemon zest, optional

Dried rose petals, optional

Flake salt, optional

Slice dates lengthwise, just enough to remove the pit but not slicing all the way through. Mix the adaptogen powder with the softened ghee, spice of your choice, and citrus zest. Once the ghee mixture is ready, take a small spoon and fill the dates with about ½ teaspoon of the mixture. Dust the stuffed dates with more citrus zest, dried rose petals, extra spices, or a sprinkle of good flake salt, and serve them on a plate. Store them in a sealed container in the fridge, if you're not enjoying immediately. They will keep for about 1 week. ■

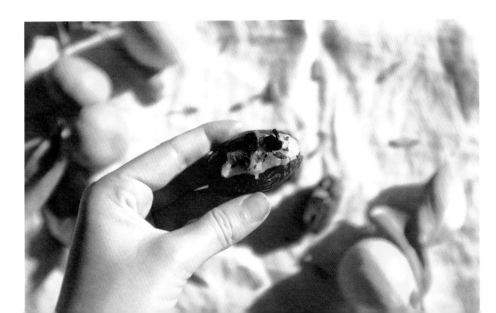

Flower Power Honey

With an abundance of flowers popping up all around, spring reminds us all to bloom and shake off the heaviness of winter. Medicinal flowers brighten any dish and often our mood. We love sprinkling fresh calendula on salads and porridge and using roses and lavender to garnish our desserts. A quick way to incorporate uplifting flower power year-round is by infusing dried flowers into an herbal honey (melita in traditional Western herbalism). You can add a spoonful of this flower-powered honey to hot tea or an herbal cocktail, drizzle it over desserts, or use it as a base for our Herbal Power Bites (page 114). FILLS 1 PINT-SIZED JAR

1 tablespoon dried calendula

1 tablespoon dried chamomile

1 tablespoon dried lavender

1 tablespoon dried rose petals

2¼ cups raw local honey

+ NOTE: All flowers should be cut and sifted.

Fill your mason jar about ⅓ to ¼ full of your favorite dried herbs, or use the measurements above as a guide. If you want it to be super potent, you can blend the dried herbs in a coffee grinder first. Pour the honey over the flowers and gently mix with the handle of a spoon or a chopstick. The more surface area of the dried herb that is submerged in the honey (or extracts in general), the more medicine will be extracted.

Allow the mixture to sit for up to 3 weeks. You can enjoy with the flowers in the mixture, or you can remove them by liquefying the honey and straining. To do this, place the closed mason jar in a pan with water that covers about ⅓ of the outside of the jar. Heat on the lowest temperature until the honey becomes smooth and liquefied. Be sure not to boil, as heating the honey too much will quickly degrade the beneficial nutrients. Pour the honey and flower mixture through a mesh strainer lined with cheesecloth into another labeled mason jar for storing and serving. Store in a cool, dark place. It will last up to 1 year if it doesn't get contaminated with food or water. To keep it fresh, it's always best to use a clean spoon each time you serve from the jar. ■

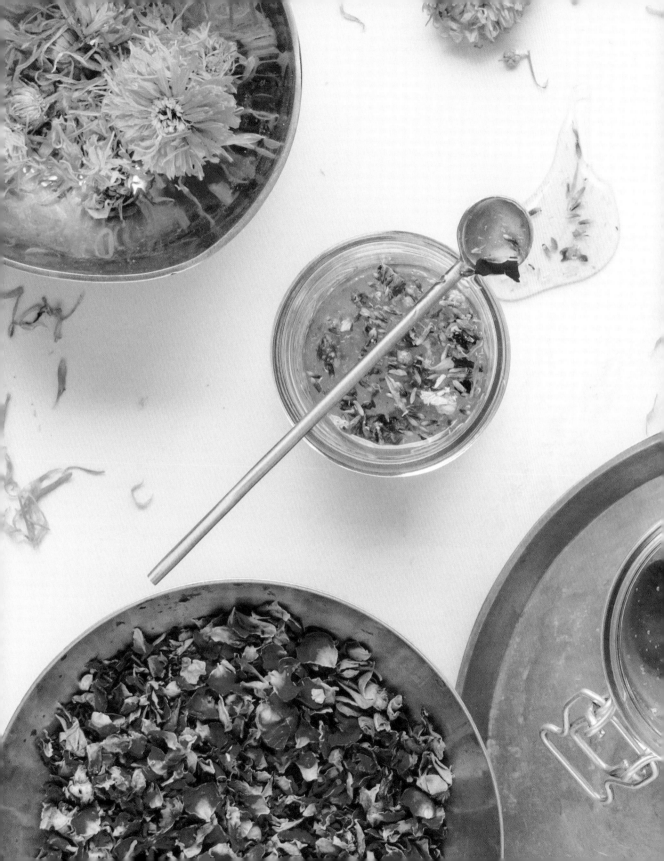

Chyawanprash Tahini Cups with Sea Salt and Rose Petals

This recipe and our Herbal Power Bites (page 114) are tasty ways to enjoy adaptogenic herbs every day. Chyawanprash (see opposite at bottom) is a rejuvenating jam from the Ayurvedic tradition that is restorative for those who are aging, run down, or anyone who wants to promote longevity and a healthy immune system.

If you want to experiment with another filling, we suggest blending soaked dates with a little sea salt and an adaptogenic powder of your choice—such as shatavari, ashwagandha, or maca—to create a gooey jam-like paste. Use this recipe as a guide and get creative with your fillings. MAKES 12 CUPS

1 cup coconut oil

1½ cups tahini

2 tablespoons maple syrup

One 8- to 12-ounce jar of chyawanprash jam

Sea salt, to taste

Dried and crushed rose petals, for garnish

Create a double boiler by placing a heat-proof stainless steel mixing bowl in a pan filled halfway with water on the stovetop, with the temperature at medium to low heat. To the bowl add the coconut oil, tahini, and maple syrup, and whisk together until smooth. Cover the bottom third (about ⅛ to ¼ inch) of each cup, lined, of a 12-count standard muffin tin with the mixture. Put the muffin tin in the freezer for 10 minutes, or until the mixture is set. Using lightly wet hands, roll a teaspoon of the chyawanprash jam into a ball, smoosh into the palm of your hand, and place on the frozen bottom tier of a muffin cup. Press down on it to flatten evenly, and leave enough space around the edges to see a circular outline of the bottom cup around the jam. Then cover the top with the remaining coconut oil and tahini mixture. Repeat with the remaining 11 cups. Finish by sprinkling each cup with sea salt and crushed rose petals. Put the cups back in the freezer for about 30 minutes or until solid. Cover and store for up to 3 months in the freezer to enjoy as a casual sweet treat. ∎

Boozy Lemon Balm Cooler

You can have a spring cooler and stay warm by using spices. This herbal refreshment uses cinnamon to promote circulation and fresh lemon balm to calm and nourish the nervous system. Make it ahead to enjoy with friends on a sunny spring day, and add simple syrup and fizzy water if you want to take it up a notch. Having a reputation among herbalists for being the bringer of gladness, lemon balm helps restore nervous system balance and soothe indigestion and anxiety. It's wonderful in teas, pesto, and infusions to brighten spirits and provide relief from melancholy. MAKES 3 CUPS

1 bottle (750 ml) of dry white wine

1 bunch (about 2 to 3 cups) fresh lemon balm

1 cinnamon stick

Edible flowers (page 70), optional

Add all the ingredients to a large glass jar or pitcher and let them infuse overnight. Strain out the herbs, chill, and enjoy. Garnish with fresh lemon balm leaves or edible flowers (page 00) of the season. ▪

TRADITIONAL FOOD: CHYAWANPRASH

This Ayurvedic medicinal jam has been used for thousands of years as a restorative formula. Known as a rasayana, it's a restorative for those who are aging or run down, and those wanting to promote longevity and a healthy immune system. One of the main herbs in this formula is called amla, also known as Indian gooseberry; it's a sour fruit packed with high levels of vitamin C. The full mix includes sugar, honey, ghee, and a mix of a few dozen herbs. This blend also stimulates the digestive system, helping it to break down and absorb essential nutrients from foods and herbs.

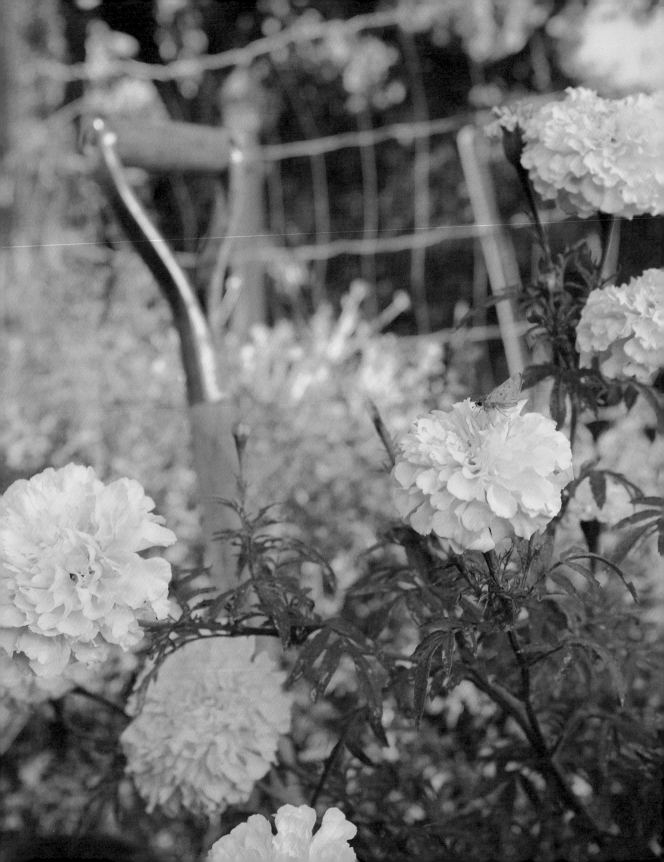

Spring Rituals for Renewal

Springtime holds a certain magic. After a long, cold winter, it's as if—all of a sudden—shades of bright green slowly awaken from their slumber and push through the moist earth. Fruiting trees are alight with their blush-colored blossoms, while the smell of sweet dew helps us breathe a little deeper and feel a little lighter. Everything is waking up and our bodies are no different. We begin to emerge from the womb of winter, ready for a fresh start.

It's important to mark each change of season with a ritual. For us, making space for ritual is a way to honor the season we're leaving and welcome the time we're entering. It's a pause in our lives to just simply be and notice what is around us. Being observant of the herbs growing around you will help guide your rituals and honor your natural rhythms during this season. Some of our favorite herbs just starting to pop up in spring happen to be wonderful supports to the lymphatic and digestive systems, helping us release some of the winter heaviness to make way for the warmer, more active months ahead. The bitter and astringent properties of many wild spring herbs support the proper digestion of fats and protein, dry excess fluids, and aid in supporting the lymphatic system's ability to remove waste from the body.

For self-care that supports these same systems, we focus on warming, stimulating, and lightly cleansing rituals to help us let go of any stagnation that has accumulated in the body over the wintertime. Here are a few of our springtime favorites.

SETTING INTENTIONS FOR GROWTH

Spring is a beautiful time to call in the things you're planting in your life to come into bloom. For us, this looks like enjoying a quiet evening at home during the first full moon of the year. Many cultures around the world mark this—the lunar New Year, as based around the thirteen full moons throughout the seasons—as the true New Year.

Your ritual for setting this intention can be anything that helps you get into the present moment. Whether that's journaling, doing breath work, or meditating, connecting with yourself is key for planting and nurturing new dreams over the next few months. If you're new to the practice of rituals, start by simply setting aside an evening to spend alone. Make yourself a nourishing dinner, take a hot bath, light candles, and listen inside yourself for what is asking to come forward. While this practice might seem simple, it truly helps us find clarity and set clear intentions for the future.

DRY BRUSHING AND SELF-OIL MASSAGE

Another ritual to help release stagnation and invite in the new season is dry brushing. This is a technique that is beneficial for supporting the lymphatic fluid that lies just below our skin, and it's an invigorating and stimulating practice that can be done daily during the cooler, moist months. Our lymph fluid doesn't have a pump like our heart does, so we must "work our lymph" by intentionally moving it. A simple way to give our lymph some extra love is by using a dry-bristle body brush to brush the skin in an upward motion toward the heart. Start at your feet and work your way up using quick strokes until you notice that your skin is pink.

Follow up the dry brushing with a self-oil massage, an ancient practice called abhyanga in Ayurveda. In the cooler months, it's best to use warming oils such as sesame to help balance the cold we're constantly feeling in our environment. This will help soothe the nervous system and keep your skin hydrated to support your precious lymphatic fluids and immune system. See page 214 for a detailed explanation of this practice.

HERBAL STEAMS: RESPIRATORY AND REPRODUCTIVE STEAMS

A steam is one of our favorite ways to use herbs for self-care. If you've ever been in a sauna, you know all about steam's relaxing and therapeutic properties. On its own, steam helps nourish, soothe, and hydrate body tissues, and can clear congested nasal passageways. By adding stimulating and nourishing herbs into the mix, steams become even more potent.

RESPIRATORY STEAM: A respiratory steam is best for when you're feeling stuffy or scratchy due to seasonal bugs or if you're looking to simply hydrate and clear up your complexion. We suggest using invigorating and soothing herbs to heal the respiratory tissues and provide some relief. The tissues in our nasal passageways are very absorbent, which allows the essential oils within these medicinal plants to quickly enter the bloodstream while you steam.

Basil	Lavender	Rosemary
Calendula	Lemon balm	Sage
Chamomile	Peppermint	Thyme
Eucalyptus	Rose	

We suggest adding 1 tablespoon each of 4 to 5 dried herbs to create a large handful. Fresh herbs will always be best, but they're not always easy to find. When using fresh herbs, you will need to add quite a bit more, about double, but just let intuition be your guide. Bring a large pot of water to boil, remove it from the heat, and then add your herbs of choice. Let the herbs steep for about 15 minutes. Get in a comfortable position, where you can place your head above the pot, and cover your head and the pot with a towel. Breathe in the steam for 10 to 15 minutes, taking breaks as needed. If you're congested, be sure to keep tissues nearby to use as your nasal passageways begin to clear.

For a more relaxing and skin-nourishing blend, use herbs such as lavender, lemon balm, calendula, chamomile, basil, and rose. If you're suffering from congestion, use invigorating herbs such as rosemary, sage, thyme, peppermint, and eucalyptus. This will help break up mucus in your nasal passageways so you can breathe easier.

Please note that eucalyptus in large quantities can be a bit too intense. We suggest using less of this herb, especially when used fresh.

Quick tip: If you're feeling pressed for time but still want the benefits of a steam, you can heat up a steamy shower and add a couple drops of a pure essential oil, such as lavender or rosemary, to the floor. The essential oils will fill the air as you shower and provide relaxation and relief.

REPRODUCTIVE STEAM: A reproductive steam, also known as a vaginal or "yoni" steam, is a wonderfully soothing practice to do once or twice a month. It helps regulate the menstrual cycle, soothes and tones vaginal tissues (especially after giving birth), reduces cysts and fibroids, aids with trauma, eases menstrual pains, increases circulation and libido, and much more. Because so much emotional energy—everything from life force and creativity to trauma—is stored in our reproductive system, this is both a physical and spiritual practice. It can be emotional, so don't be surprised if you feel a wave of release and shed some tears throughout the process.

+ SAFETY: Please do not do a reproductive steam if you're currently bleeding or pregnant, have an IUD, an infection, or open wounds. If you have any ongoing reproductive challenges, it's best to consult with an herbal practitioner or health-care provider before use.

Basil	Motherwort	Rose
Calendula	Mugwort	Rosemary
Chamomile	Plantain	Yarrow
Lavender	Raspberry leaf	

We suggest using about 1 cup total of dried herbs for your reproductive steam; if you're using fresh herbs, double the amount (approximately; lightly chopped) and let intuition guide you. Add your herbs to a pot and pour boiling water over them. Allow the mixture to cool slightly and place it under a slatted wooden chair or a stool made for yoni steams, or place it in a bowl and put inside a clean toilet so you can sit over it.

The closer you are to the pot, the more you will need the mixture to cool down, so the steam doesn't burn you as you're sitting over it. You want it to be warm but not at all uncomfortable. It may take up to 5 to 10 minutes to cool and become comfortable; stay patient, as you're working with very tender tissues. Wear socks and cover your neck and body with blankets, wrapping the blankets around you to help trap in the warmth of the steam. We suggest dropping into a meditation or listening to soothing music. Take about 20 to 30 minutes for this practice. Afterward, keep covered to stay warm and grounded. This is a cleansing ritual, so it's best to stay hydrated and nourished afterward by drinking plenty of water and avoiding alcohol. Take it easy for the day and stay gentle with yourself.

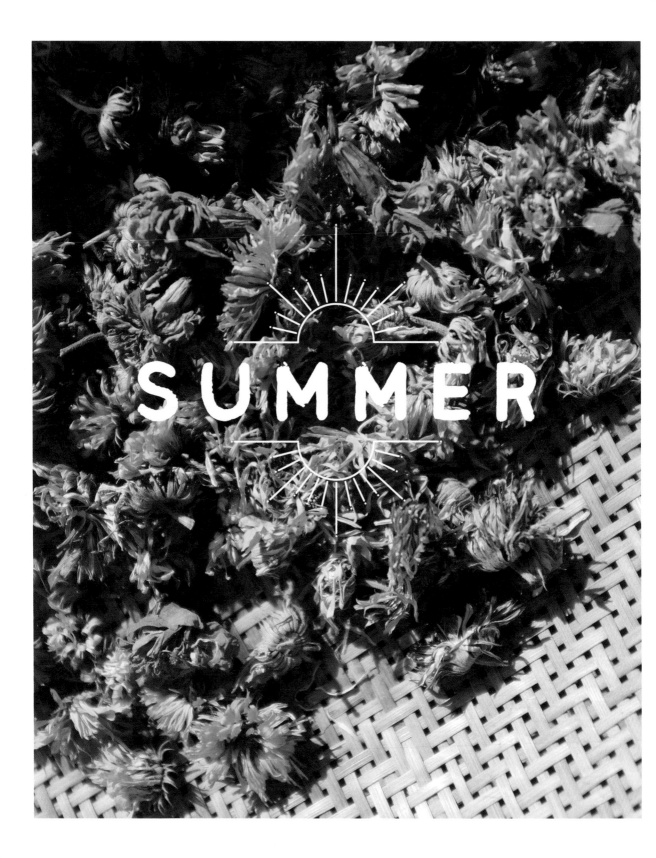

SUMMER

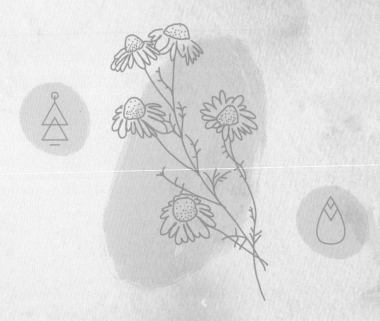

THE FIERY NATURE OF SUMMER BRINGS US ULTIMATE GROWTH and abundance. It's a time of expansion, blossoming, and becoming. It's when our gardens are most abundant, and when all that manifestation and ritual work we did in winter and spring finally comes to fruition. Summer is when all of our personal growth leads us to transformation.

With long, sunny days and frequent gatherings, we can feel so energized that we end up overcommitting. It's possible to have a little too much fun, and we need to rest, restore, and cool down. This is why herbalists tend to use cooling herbs such as aloe, hibiscus, peppermint, and lemon balm during this season. Summer can be dry or wet, depending on your ecosystem. If your climate is drier, focus on using hydrating mucilaginous plants such as oats and marshmallow root, and eating foods that are sweet, milky, and restorative—creamy foods such as ghee, soup, and porridge. If it's wet where you live, consume less milky foods and focus more on bitter and astringent herbs and foods, including greens such as dandelion and arugula, and more raw foods. If you tend to run on the colder side naturally, enjoying warming peppers and nightshades shouldn't be a problem this time of year.

This heated season is more active, so like a pitta person, you likely will have more energy. It's a good time to wake up early, stay active, and finish early to escape the heat and calm the mind. Create a manageable schedule for yourself, so you don't overdo it, and engage in rituals that support your digestive and nervous systems.

FOODS	HERBS	RITUALS	REDUCE
Raw, light, bitter and cooling foods, such as sprouts, salads, and veggies Topping meals with lots of cooling and soothing fresh green herbs, such as basil, cilantro, mint, and parsley Naturally sweet foods, such as fresh seasonal fruits, grains, moderate dairy, and root vegetables	Cooling herbs and spices: aloe, basil, cilantro, coriander, cumin, dandelion greens, dill, fennel, mint, parsley, turmeric Calming nervous system herbs: catnip, chamomile, hops, lavender, lemon balm, oats, passionflower, skullcap Cooling and moistening adaptogens: licorice, reishi, shatavari	Breath work Meditation Swimming Abhyanga (page 214), with cooling oils, such as coconut, and calming essential oils, such as lavender and chamomile Restorative yoga Long walks	Salty, sour, spicy, pungent tastes Oily foods, such as olives and nuts, and fried foods Nightshades, such as onions, eggplant, and tomatoes Chocolate, acidic foods, and alcohol Overworking to the point of burnout

SUMMER SEASON

ELEMENTS: Fire and water

QUALITIES: Hot and wet

DOSHA: Pitta

BALANCING SUMMER FLAVORS: Astringent, bitter, sweet

SIGNALS OF BALANCE: Feeling cool and calm, driven, optimistic, passionate, taking breaks rather than pushing through, staying hydrated and nourished

SIGNALS OF IMBALANCE: Feeling hot and inflamed, hot-tempered, easily frustrated, overworking yourself, allergic reactions, regular headaches, rashes, acidic digestion, and loose stool

Everyday Summer Brew

During the hot days of summer, having a refreshing tea is a daily necessity to stay hydrated and nourished. Here in the Mediterranean climate of Northern California, summers get incredibly dry and hot. It's easy to get out of balance and end up feeling depleted, irritated, and burned out during the summer months. One of our favorite ways to make sure we're supporting our hydration is by brewing a large jar of tea each evening to enjoy the next day.

To make your tea ritual simple, the key is to mix a weekly batch of your favorite dried herbal tea blend to save time and encourage you to drink about a quart of tea each day. The amounts we provide in this recipe will make about a pint-sized mason jar of this herbal blend, so you can have it handy to enjoy throughout the week.

Fresh herbs are in abundance this time of year, so we encourage you to use what you can find or grow in your garden, along with any dried herbs. Some of our favorite herbs with bitter, cooling, and calming properties are mint, chamomile, and lemon balm. We added marshmallow root to this blend for its moistening and cooling properties. But if you live in a more tropical place, substitute tulsi, which is more drying, to help balance the excess moisture.

FILLS 1 PINT-SIZED JAR

½ **cup dried lemon balm**

¼ **cup dried mint**

¼ **cup dried chamomile**

¼ **cup dried passionflower**

½ **cup dried marshmallow root**

+ NOTE: **All herbs and flowers should be cut and sifted.**

Add all the herbs to a mixing bowl and mix to combine, or just add them directly to the jar, leaving a little space at the top so you can close the lid and shake to combine.

To make a daily quart of tea, add 2 to 3 tablespoons of the tea blend to a quart-sized mason jar. Fill the jar with cold water, leaving about 1 inch of room at the top. Close the lid and put in the fridge to infuse overnight. The tea will be ready in the morning to strain through a mesh strainer or French press. Store the strained tea in a mason jar to carry with you throughout the day or keep in the fridge for up to 2 days. We suggest drinking a quart a day, or at least 2 to 3 cups to get the most benefit. Pour yourself a glass whenever you want to wind down and relax, or even shake with ice to create a summer cooler. ∎

Lavender, Chamomile, and Skullcap Cooler

At the height of the summer, we often find ourselves committing to far too much. The long, bright days inspire us to work and play a little harder than we probably should. This herbal cooler is the perfect summer remedy and will inspire you take it down a notch.

This cooler has chamomile and lavender to calm the mind and belly, and skullcap to actively soothe and tonify the nervous system. FILLS 1 QUART-SIZED JAR

2 tablespoons dried chamomile

1 teaspoon dried lavender

1 tablespoon dried skullcap

2 tablespoons raw local honey or sweetener of choice

4 cups water

Juice of 2 lemons

Lemon slices, optional

Lavender sprigs, optional

Edible flowers (page 70)

+ NOTE: If you tend to run cold and want to warm up this blend, grate in a bit of fresh ginger to taste.

+ NOTE: All herbs and flowers should be cut and sifted.

Add your dried herbs to a glass quart-sized mason jar. Boil the water and pour it into the jar. If the temperature inside is cool, make sure to preheat the jar to prevent the glass from breaking. Cover with the lid and allow the mixture to steep for 15 to 20 minutes. Add in the honey or sweetener of choice and stir to dissolve. Give it a taste to check the sweetness and adjust if necessary. Once cool, add in the lemon juice and store in the fridge. Serve chilled, and garnish with thin lemon slices and sprigs of lavender or fresh edible flowers. ■

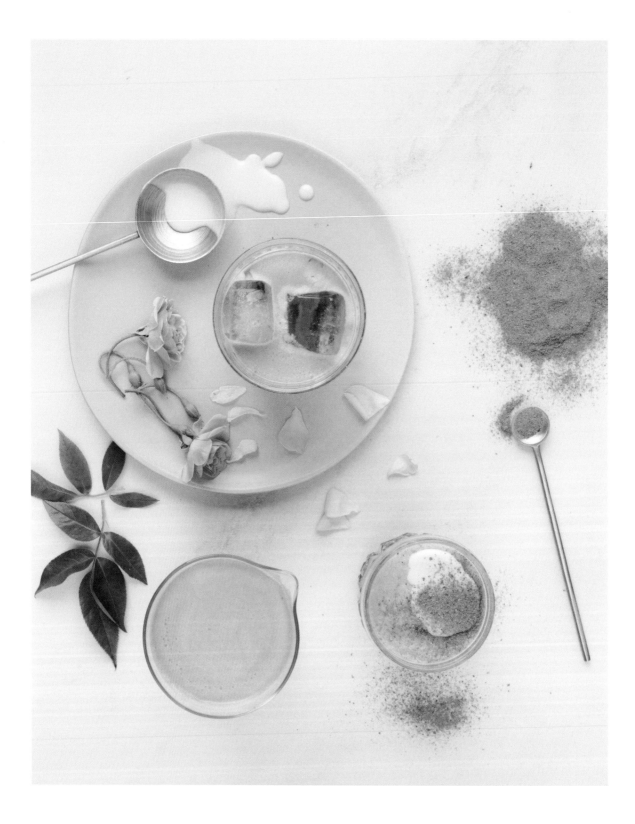

Kava Kava White Russian

Who needs alcohol when you can have herbs instead? While we will have a boozy drink on occasion, we usually opt for calming and heart-opening herbs such as kava kava. This sacred root (see below) is known for its mouth-numbing effect, so don't be alarmed if you have a temporary tingly feeling. This means it's working. Try serving this at an intimate gathering and set a collective intention for the night. Emotions may flow, as this plant is known to open up the heart for healthy communication.

+ SAFETY: As this plant is powerful and can get you fairly buzzed, we recommend not consuming more than 1 to 2 cups. As with any sedative, it's best to not drive after drinking too much or abuse its powers over time.

SERVES 2 TO 3

One 13.5-ounce can full-fat coconut milk or homemade nut milk (page 90)

1 to 2 tablespoons powdered kava kava

½ teaspoon ground cinnamon, plus more for serving

½ teaspoon ground cardamom

1 cup coffee, can be decaf or an herbal "coffee" option

4 to 5 tablespoons maple syrup

1 pinch sea salt

Crushed rose petals, for garnish

The night before, add the coconut milk, powdered kava kava, cinnamon, and cardamom to a quart-sized mason jar and cover, allowing the mixture to infuse overnight. The next day, strain out the herbs using a mesh strainer lined with cheesecloth.

Combine the coconut milk mixture, coffee, and maple syrup and add back to the jar along with a pinch of salt. Add ice, cover, and shake to combine, then pour each serving over a large single ice cube to serve. You can add a touch of water to the mix if it feels too thick. Garnish with ground cinnamon and crushed rose petals and serve immediately. ■

TRADITIONAL HERB: KAVA KAVA

Kava kava (Piper methysticum) is a sacred plant from the Fijian islands/ Oceania that is traditionally used in ceremonies to honor life or death, resolve conflict, offer hospitality, and more. Each region has their own practices and history surrounding this precious medicinal root. In modern times, you may see kava bars or people consuming it for ongoing anxiety. It's best used in personal or communal ceremony, with clear intentions in mind. Try focusing on a certain result or theme and enjoying a more relaxed and meditative state.

Hibiscus Punch with Schisandra Salt Rims

This is one of our favorite summertime drinks that brings us back to our time in Oaxaca, Mexico. Hibiscus, also known as *jamaica* in Mexico, is cooling and astringent in nature, which makes an ideal beverage for hot and humid climates. Dried hibiscus is actually the calyx, or collective sepals, that serves as a base to the flower as it's in bloom and is left when the flower falls off. Plants that are high in vitamin C, such as hibiscus, are best extracted in cold water, so this will be an overnight cold brew. To make this drink more special, we give it a salt rim with a flavor-rich adaptogen, schisandra berry powder. This punch is made as a concentrate, so it can be enjoyed alone, with sparkling water, or with a splash of something boozy, such as a smoky mezcal. FILLS 1 QUART-SIZED JAR

1 cup dried hibiscuss

2 cinnamon sticks

4 cups water

1 to 2 tablespoons raw local honey

1 tablespoon sea salt

1 tablespoon schisandra berry powder

1 lime, cut into wedges

Ice, optional

Sparkling water, optional

Mezcal, optional

Edible flowers (page 70), optional

Add the hibiscus and cinnamon sticks to a quart-sized mason jar and fill with the water. Cover with a tight lid and let sit in the fridge overnight. Strain the concentrate using a mesh strainer or French press and pour into a quart-sized mason jar. In a small bowl, thin the honey with a splash or two of warm water so it mixes easier with the punch. Stir in the honey and taste, adjusting sweetness to your liking.

Mix the sea salt and schisandra berry powder together in a small bowl, then pour in an even layer onto a small plate. Use a lime wedge to swirl around the rim of a glass, then dip the rim into the salt mix. Repeat with the other glasses.

To serve, fill the glasses with ice cubes, if using, and pour in the concentrate for a strong punch. Alternatively, you can use a shaker to cool the concentrate down, then add a splash of sparkling water or mezcal, if you like. Add a squeeze of fresh lime and top with a few edible flower petals for garnish. ■

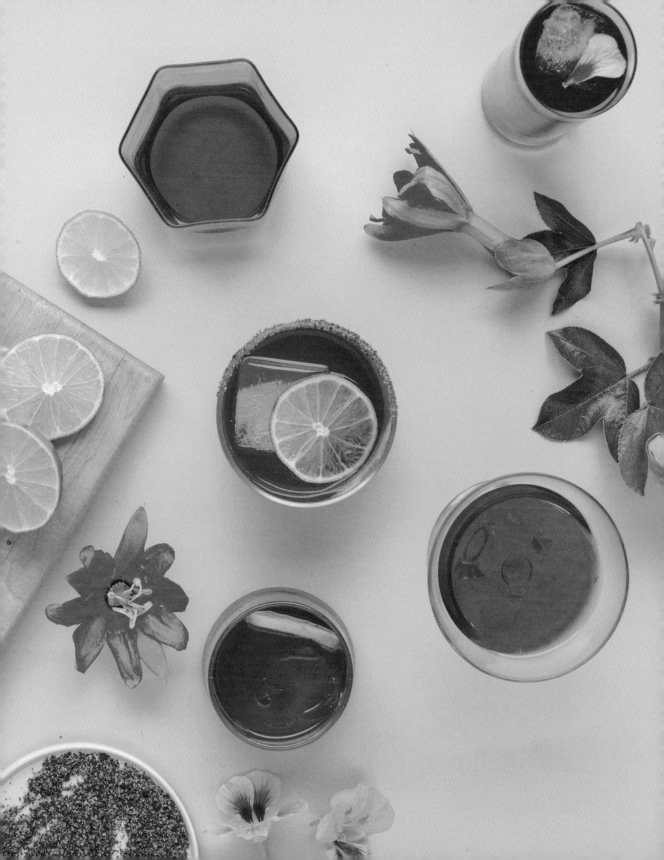

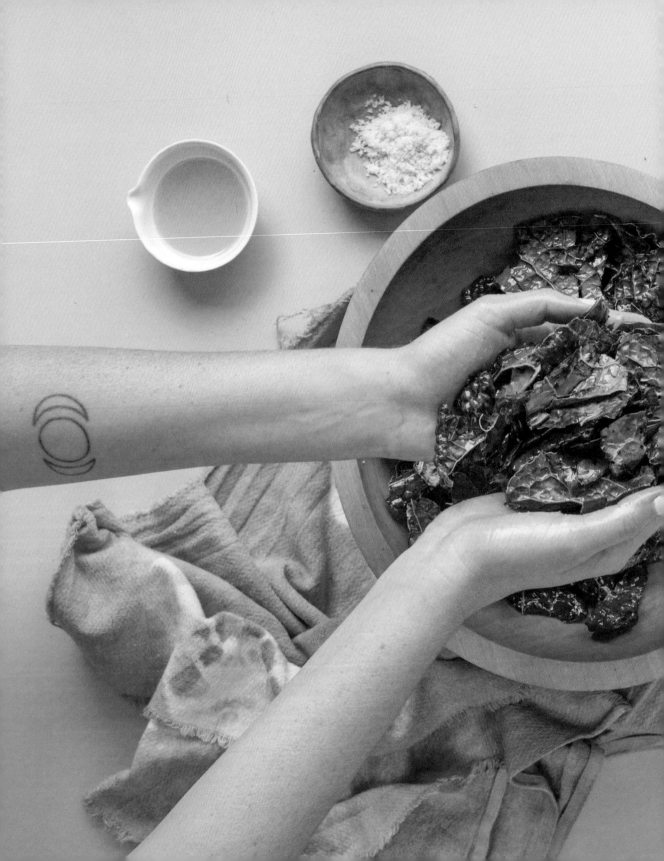

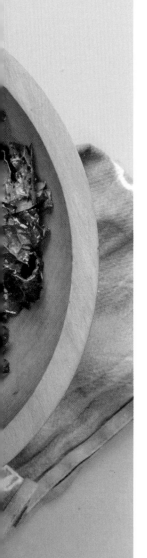

Magical Massaged Kale Breakfast Bowl

There's a reason they say breakfast is the most important meal of the day. Having something within the first two hours of waking helps support healthy hormone levels and ensures your day starts off with a burst of energy. Protein is an important part of this nourishing breakfast equation. Whether that's a runny egg, smoked salmon, tempeh, or beans, protein is the ideal fuel for the morning.

The key to this recipe is having your staples on hand: cooked grains, herbal pesto or dressing, and toasted seeds. With these already made, this savory breakfast bowl can be made in minutes and is sure to satisfy when you need something substantial on a summer morning. SERVES 2

2 cups cooked grains, such as rice or quinoa

1 tablespoon Ghee (page 110) or coconut oil

1 garlic clove, smashed and minced

1 bunch kale, rinsed, de-stemmed, and torn into bite-sized pieces

½ tablespoon olive oil, plus more for garnish

Pinch of sea salt and black pepper

Squeeze of fresh lemon juice

2 tablespoons Wild Weeds Pesto (page 102) or dressing

6 ounces protein, such as smoked salmon, runny egg, or tempeh

¼ cup toasted nuts or seeds

Flake salt, for garnish

Start by reheating your grain on the stove. Melt the ghee in a pan on medium-low heat, then add in the garlic, cooking until fragrant but not browned. Toss in your grain and stir to coat, then let it sit undisturbed to form a crunchy bottom while you get the kale ready. All types of kale or hearty greens can work in this recipe, but our favorite has to be lacinato kale, also known as dinosaur kale. Put the kale in a large mixing bowl and add the olive oil, salt, and fresh lemon juice on top. Start massaging the kale with your hands, squeezing to soften the leaves. Do this for a few minutes, or until the raw kale is tender to your liking. Taste and adjust with more salt or lemon juice.

By this time, your grain should be warm, crispy, and ready to remove from the heat. Season the grain with salt and pepper, then divide evenly between two bowls. Dollop 1 tablespoon of pesto or herbal dressing onto the grain, nestle in your protein, then top with a handful of the massaged kale and the toasted nuts or seeds. We also like to add a pinch of flake salt and an extra drizzle of olive oil for good measure. ■

Buckwheat Crepes with Raspberries and Cashew Cream

Buckwheat crepes are so simple to make, and the toppings can be tailored to fit any season. In the summertime we like to keep it simple with a little sugar, lemon, and fresh fruits of the season. Come winter, we top them with savory herbs, eggs, and roasted veggies. See the crepe as a vehicle for whatever herbs and foods you're feeling called to, based on the season or your dosha. These crepes are perfect to share as a group, because everyone can flavor their plate their own way. MAKES ABOUT 10 CREPES

2 eggs

¾ teaspoon sea salt

1 cup buckwheat flour

1 cup milk of choice

1 tablespoon butter, Ghee (page 110), or coconut oil

TOPPINGS

Cashew Cream (recipe follows)

Summer berries, such as blackberries, blueberries, and/or raspberries

Brown sugar or raw local honey, to taste

Edible flowers (page 70), such as borage, calendula, and chamomile, for garnish

3 lemons, sliced in quarters

First, make sure you have a crepe pan or large pan and a big spatula. In a small bowl, mix the eggs together with a hand whisk. In a large mixing bowl, mix together the sea salt and flour, then whisk in the eggs, and then the milk. The batter will look really thin, which is what you want. Cover the mixture and put it in the fridge while prepping your topping ingredients or even overnight to prep breakfast for the next day.

When you're ready to make the crepes, take the batter out of the fridge and mix in a touch more water to thin it out, if needed. Put the crepe pan over medium heat and add the butter, to keep the batter from sticking to the pan. Pour in about a ¼ cup of batter, or enough to fill the shape of the pan, per crepe. Cook each side of the crepe for 1 to 2 minutes, until golden in hue. Stack and cover the crepes with kitchen towels so they stay warm. Then serve with your toppings of choice. For the summer, we recommend spreading the cashew cream across half the crepe and topping with fresh berries, brown sugar, and edible flowers. Before serving, squeeze fresh lemon juice over the crepes.

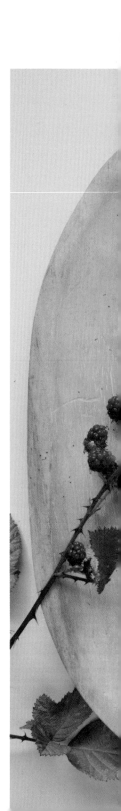

Cashew Cream

1 cup raw cashews

½ cup water

½ tablespoon maple syrup

1 teaspoon ground cinnamon

Juice of ½ to 1 lemon

½ teaspoon sea salt, to taste

Begin by soaking the cashews, making sure they are covered by an inch or so of water for at least 1 hour, or overnight if possible. Strain, and to a high-powered blender add the cashews, water, maple syrup, cinnamon, lemon juice, and a pinch of sea salt. Blend until creamy, like ricotta or even a bit smoother.

+ TIP: If you want to create a savory version, simply omit the maple syrup and cinnamon and substitute with lemon juice and freshly chopped herbs such as basil and chives. This will give the cream a savory finish, and you can use it as a base for eggs and sautéed veggies or on our Magical Massaged Kale Breakfast Bowl (page 159). You can also combine it with the Wild Weeds Pesto (page 102) or drizzle the creamy Turmeric Tahini Dressing (page 105) on top of your crepe, cashew cream, and greens. ■

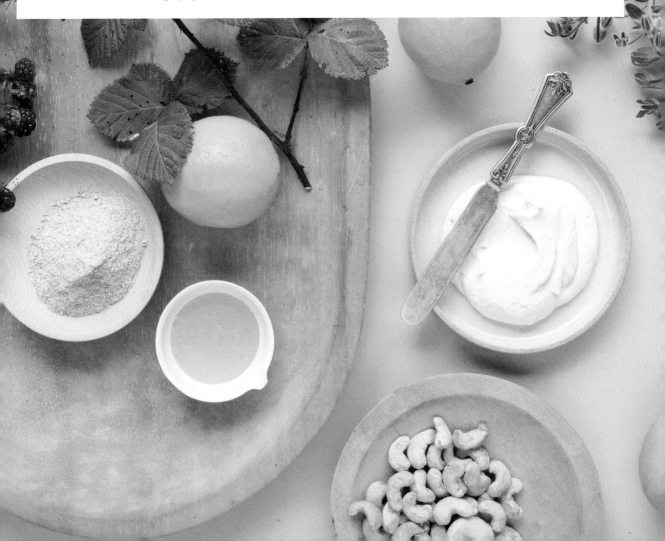

Buckwheat Soba Salad with Turmeric Tahini Dressing

This salad can be enjoyed as a main dish or part of a summer picnic spread. There's something so satisfying about the nuttiness from the buckwheat noodles tossed with crunchy vegetables and a creamy dressing. The Turmeric Tahini Dressing is one of our most-loved recipes and a staple in many of our students' kitchens. It has the perfect amount of sweet and savory notes, and the garlic and turmeric support the immune system and promote circulation—a perfect duo to support the body during the transitions between seasons. This dressing can be used in the heat of summer with raw crunchy veggies and soba noodles, or in a warm winter salad with rice and massaged leafy greens or roasted vegetables. SERVES 4

8 to 10 ounces buckwheat soba noodles

2 red bell peppers

1 to 2 jalapenos, deseeded

¼ purple cabbage

1 cup Turmeric Tahini Dressing (page 105)

4 tablespoons black sesame seeds

1 teaspoon dulse seaweed flakes

½ bunch cilantro, about 1 cup

Pinch of sea salt, to taste

Juice of 1 lime

Cook noodles according to the package directions, then strain and rinse them with cold water, allowing them to cool. While the noodles cook, deseed the red bell peppers and cut them lengthwise. Use a mandolin to slice the red bell pepper into long thin strips. Slice the jalapeno in thin half-moon shapes using a knife. Use a mandolin to cut thin slices of cabbage. Set the vegetables aside. In a big bowl, toss the noodles in the dressing and slowly add in the chopped veggies. We use enough dressing to make it runny, like a slaw. Top with the black sesame seeds, seaweed flakes, and cilantro. Dress with a sprinkle of sea salt and a squeeze of fresh lime juice. ■

Melon, Tomato, and Mint Salad

This recipe is ridiculously simple and indescribably delicious. You will have all of your guests asking for the recipe, as this olive oil–infused fruit salad is both unique and so refreshing. It's inspired by Summer's time studying abroad in Spain, where she learned about the magical combination of fresh tomatoes, honeydew melon, olive oil, and salt from her gracious host mom María José. We love including fresh mint to add some extra flavor and cooling energy in the heat of the summer season. The longer this salad has to marinate during the day, the better it becomes. It's perfect for sunny summer picnics and cookouts. SERVES 4

1 honeydew melon

1 dry pint (about 1½ cups) cherry tomatoes

4 tablespoons olive oil

1 teaspoon sea salt, or more to taste

3 to 4 sprigs of fresh mint

Cut the rind off the melon and slice it into 1-inch cubes. Slice the cherry tomatoes in half. In a large mixing bowl, add the melon, tomatoes, olive oil, and salt, and mix to combine. Let the salad sit for at least 20 to 30 minutes so the fruits can soak up all the flavor. If it's cool inside, you can leave the mixture covered right on the countertop. If it's hot, cover the bowl and place it in the fridge to marinate. Finely chop the fresh mint leaves and garnish the salad before serving. ■

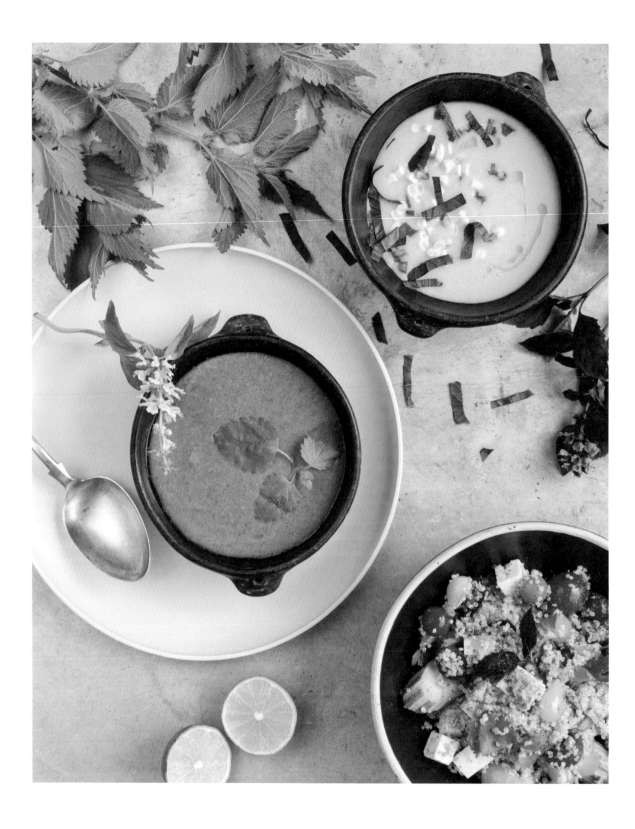

Lemon Balm Gazpacho with Za'atar Quinoa and Cucumber Salad

When it's too hot to cook, nothing beats the refreshing flavor of a blended soup heavy on fresh herbs. Lemon balm has a sweet citrus scent and slightly bitter flavor to help keep us cool, support our nervous system, and aid in soothing digestive woes. While it's generally used to flavor tea, its lemony flavor is a perfect complement to this twist on a traditional gazpacho.

To make a full meal, this quick quinoa salad does the trick. If you're not familiar with za'atar, you'll soon want to put it on everything from salads and roasted vegetables to eggs. You can easily make your own, but the blend can also be found in herb shops and specialty markets. SERVES 4

Lemon Balm Gazpacho

2 handfuls (about 3 cups) fresh lemon balm leaves

¼ cup fresh mint leaves, chopped

2 cucumbers, deseeded and chopped

1 yellow bell pepper, deseeded and chopped

1 avocado, peeled and pit removed

2 garlic cloves, smashed

½ tablespoon white wine vinegar or lemon juice

1 pinch ground cayenne

1 teaspoon sea salt

½ cup water; use less if you want a thicker gazpacho

Edible flowers (page 70), optional

Olive oil, optional

In a high-speed blender, add all the ingredients and blend until smooth. Taste and adjust the mint, garlic, or vinegar ratios to your liking. Store the soup in a mason jar and let it cool in the fridge before serving. To serve, make this extra-special by topping with fresh edible flowers and a drizzle of good olive oil.

recipe continues on following page

Quinoa and Cucumber Salad

1 tablespoon za'atar (see below)

2 tablespoons fresh lemon juice

¼ cup olive oil

Sea salt and fresh cracked black pepper

4 cups cooked quinoa, room temperature

1 cup chopped fresh parsley or basil, reserving 1 tablespoon for garnish

2 cups cherry tomatoes, halved

1 cucumber, deseeded and skin partially peeled in long strips

1 cup feta cheese, cubed or crumbled

FOR THE DRESSING: In a small bowl, whisk the za'atar with the lemon juice while drizzling in the olive oil so it emulsifies into a silky dressing. Taste and add a pinch of sea salt and black pepper, then set aside so the flavors have a chance to marinate.

FOR THE SALAD: In a large mixing bowl, add the quinoa, chopped herbs, tomatoes, and cucumber, tossing to combine. Pour over the dressing a few spoonfuls at a time and toss well. Just before serving, sprinkle over the feta, an extra drizzle of olive oil, and reserved herbs for garnish. ■

ZA'ATAR

To make your own za'atar spice mix, combine 1 tablespoon each of dried oregano, sumac, sesame seeds, and cumin in a small bowl or jar. Then add 1 teaspoon each of sea salt and freshly cracked black pepper. Store in a small glass jar with a tight-fitting lid to maintain freshness.

Sweet Corn and Coconut Soup with Jalapeno-Nettle Pistou

Fresh sweet corn is a highlight of the summer market. While it's satisfying simply grilled, one of our favorite ways to enjoy its sweetness is in a soup made creamy with russet potatoes and coconut milk. To help balance the sweetness, a drizzle of our mineral-rich pistou adds a spicy kick. Pistou is a Provençal sauce usually made with basil, olive oil, garlic, and salt; it's similar to pesto without the traditional pine nuts. You'll probably want to make extra pistou so you'll have it on hand for grilled vegetables, salad dressings, or mixing into grains throughout the week. If you have any leftover soup, simply store in the fridge and serve chilled for lunch the next day. SERVES 2 TO 3

1 tablespoon Ghee (page 110) or coconut oil

1 yellow onion, diced

½ teaspoon ground turmeric

1 russet potato, cut into small cubes

5 ears fresh sweet corn, kernels removed, ½ cup reserved for garnish

6 cups Everyday Herbal Bone Broth (page 112), vegetable broth, or water

1½ teaspoons sea salt

One 13.5-ounce can or 1½ cups full-fat coconut milk

Juice of 2 limes

Jalapeno-Nettle Pistou (recipe follows)

In a heavy-bottomed soup pot on medium heat, melt your fat and add the onion, cooking until soft and translucent, but making sure the onions don't brown. Next, add in the turmeric, potatoes, and corn, stirring to combine. Pour in the broth, season with sea salt, and bring to a simmer. Let the soup cook until the vegetables are softened, about 15 to 20 minutes. Turn off the heat and stir in the coconut milk and fresh lime juice. Using an immersion blender, blend the soup until smooth and creamy. If you don't have an immersion blender, you can add the soup in batches to a high-speed blender and blend until creamy. If it needs more liquid, add in water, broth, or coconut milk ¼ cup at a time to thin it out to your liking. To serve, ladle the soup into bowls and top each with a drizzle of the Jalapeno-Nettle Pistou and reserved corn kernels.

recipe continues on following page

Jalapeno–Nettle Pistou

MAKES ABOUT 1 CUP

2 cups roughly chopped fresh
nettle leaves

2 garlic cloves, minced

1 jalapeno, deseeded and chopped

2 cups roughly chopped sweet
basil leaves

Juice of 2 limes

¼ teaspoon sea salt

¾ cup olive oil

Fill a saucepan about halfway with water, cover, and bring to a boil. While waiting for the water to boil, make an ice bath by filling a prep bowl halfway with ice and water. Once the water is boiling, toss in the chopped nettle leaves and blanch for about 10 seconds. This will help soften the nettle and make it easier to create a smooth texture for the pistou. Using a mesh sieve or colander, strain the nettle leaves and sit the strainer in the ice bath for about 1 minute. Remove the strainer with the nettle and press out any excess water over the sink with the back of a wooden spoon or by wrapping tightly in a kitchen towel. In a food processor, add all the ingredients and pulse until smooth. If you have a food processor that has the attachment to drizzle in the olive oil as the rest of the ingredients are blending, that will help the pistou emulsify better. Taste and add more salt or lime juice to your liking. Pour into a small mason jar with a tight-fitting lid and store in the fridge until ready to serve. Use within 3 days. ∎

CORN SILK

Fresh corn in the height of summer should have bright shiny silks. Corn silk is a cooling diuretic and is a wonderful medicine to soothe the mucous membranes of the urinary system. You can make a strong tea by boiling 1 quart of water and steeping about 1 cup of corn silk for 20 minutes. Sip throughout the day to ease inflammation from dehydration.

Summer Dips: Tulsi Pesto and Red Pepper Muhammara

On days when it's just too hot to cook, making a snack board to enjoy midday does the trick. By simply slicing fresh vegetables, arranging crackers, and making a quick dip or two, lunch is served with little effort and without using the stove. This is also a great option for easy summer entertaining. We used to make pesto with tulsi when we had an abundance in our garden in Orlando, and it was always a hit. It has a really lovely flavor that's reminiscent of its cousin sweet basil but with a spicy edge. These two dips make a regular appearance in our kitchens because we usually have the ingredients on hand and they're a breeze to make. Double the recipe to make a big batch to enjoy throughout the week.

Tulsi Pesto

MAKES ABOUT 2 CUPS

1 cup nuts or seeds of choice, soaked overnight and strained (see page 90)

2 to 3 garlic cloves

¼ teaspoon sea salt, or more to taste

2 cups packed fresh mix of tulsi, sweet basil, and/or cilantro

Juice of 1 lemon

¾ cup extra virgin olive oil

Add the nuts or seeds and garlic to a food processor and pulse until it resembles a course meal. Sprinkle in sea salt, then add the fresh basil. Squeeze in the fresh lemon juice, then add half of the olive oil. Pulse again to incorporate, then leave the motor going while drizzling in the rest of the olive oil, until the pesto is nice and creamy. Taste and adjust salt, lemon, or olive oil to your liking. Store in a wide-mouth jar, drizzling a little more oil to cover the top of the pesto. This will help prevent any browning or oxidization that can occur on top. Store in the fridge with a well-sealed lid to stay fresh for up to a week.

recipe continues on following page

Red Pepper Muhammara

MAKES ABOUT 2 CUPS

1 cup walnuts, toasted

One 12-ounce jar roasted red
peppers, skins removed

1 tablespoon pomegranate molasses

½ tablespoon fresh lemon juice

1 teaspoon ground cumin

1 garlic clove

½ teaspoon sea salt

¼ cup olive oil

Edible flowers (page 70), optional

Add walnuts to a food processor and lightly pulse, until they have a crumbly consistency. Strain the red peppers well and pat dry with a clean dish towel. This will help avoid a watery dip. Add them to the food processor along with all the other ingredients. Pulse the mixture until smooth. Add more olive oil if you desire a creamier dip, and taste and adjust the lemon juice and salt to your liking.

Serve with pita chips, sliced vegetables, or over grains for added flavor. You can also garnish the dip with fresh edible flowers such as calendula, borage, pansies, or whatever is seasonally handy. ■

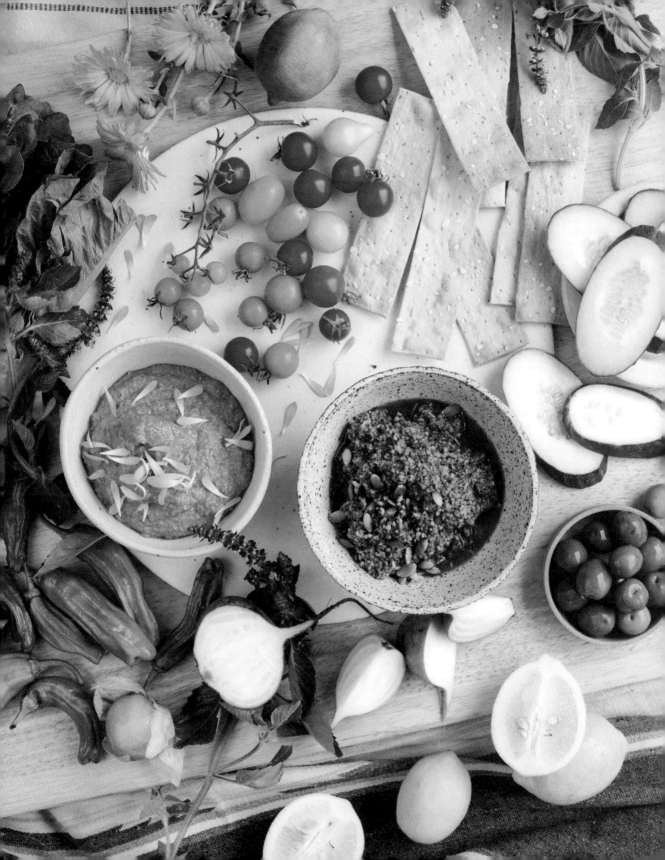

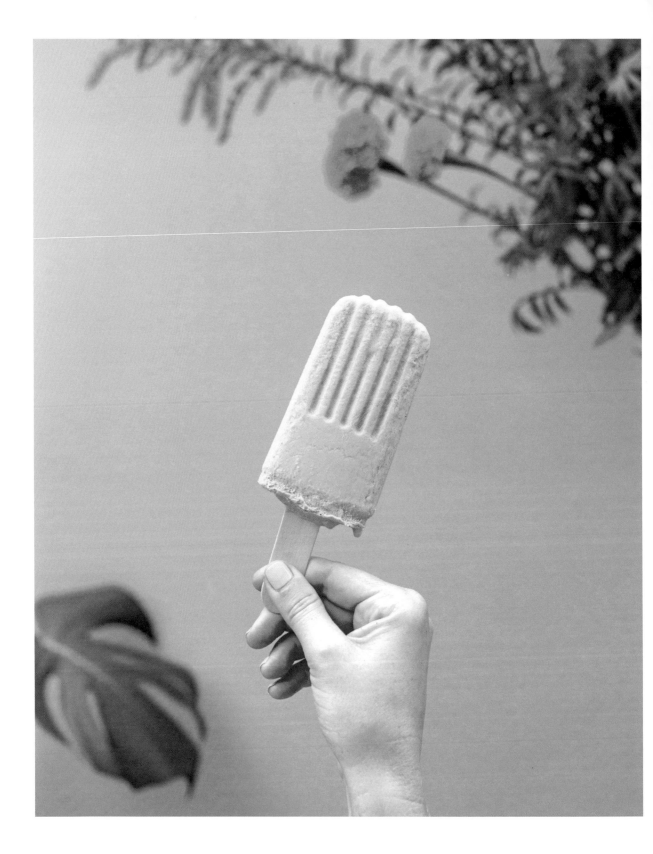

Coco Golden Milk Pops

We're usually not fans of cold foods and drinks because they tend to put out our digestive fire. But every once in a while, especially on a hot summer day, enjoying an herbal popsicle is the only way to beat the heat. These pops are a riff off of everyone's favorite tonic beverage, golden milk. Adding the warming spices of black pepper and cardamom, and the slightly bitter flavor of turmeric, helps to balance the fact that these are frozen.

You might be surprised to see chia seeds in popsicles, but they're one of our favorite foods to enjoy this time of year since they help us stay hydrated with their moistening quality. These small but mighty seeds, indigenous to the pre-Columbian Mesoamerican cultures, are high in magnesium, omega-3 fatty acids, and antioxidants. For a refreshing summer drink, try adding 1 tablespoon of chia seeds to a quart of water or fresh pressed juice. MAKES 6 MILK POPS

+ SPECIAL EQUIPMENT: **Steel popsicle molds**

Two 13.5-ounce cans or 2¼ cups full-fat coconut milk

1 tablespoon chia seeds

1 teaspoon turmeric powder

1 teaspoon ground cardamom

Pinch of finely ground black pepper

3 tablespoons maple syrup

Mix the coconut milk and chia seeds in a bowl or jar and let sit for about 10 minutes to hydrate the chia seeds. You'll know the chia seeds are ready when they've become plump. Next, add the chia mixture, turmeric, cardamom, black pepper, and maple syrup to a high-speed blender and blend on low until combined. Taste and adjust the sweetness to your liking. Pour the mixture evenly into the popsicle molds, place a stick in each one, and put the molds in the freezer to set. Once the pops have frozen, they can be removed from the molds by running them under warm water until they release. ■

Summer Berry Crumble with Chamomile and Lavender Coconut Cream

We recommend sourcing the freshest summer berries you can find for this: blueberries, strawberries, raspberries, or blackberries all work wonderfully. The chamomile and lavender coconut cream complement the berries and their naturally tart flavor. This sweet and relaxing topping also goes well on lattes, mousses, and fresh fruit. Both recipes can be made ahead of time and stored in the fridge and reheated for summer gatherings. SERVES 6

½ cup plus 1 teaspoon coconut oil, divided

Two 16-ounce cartons fresh strawberries, or 4 cups seasonal berries of choice, roughly chopped

Juice of ½ lemon

1 cup rolled oats

¼ cup brown or coconut sugar

½ cup walnuts

½ cup sunflower seeds

1½ tablespoons maca powder

½ teaspoon ground cardamom powder

½ teaspoon sea salt

½ teaspoon poppy seeds, optional

Chamomile and Lavender Coconut Cream (recipe follows)

Preheat oven to 350°F. Grease a medium-sized baking dish with 1 teaspoon coconut oil and add the strawberries in an even layer. Squeeze the lemon juice over the freshly chopped fruit. In a food processor, combine the oats, sugar, walnuts, sunflower seeds, ½ cup coconut oil, maca powder (or neutral tasting) adaptogen powder choice, cardamom, and sea salt. Pulse a few times until a very rough crumble forms. Test the texture of the crumble by pinching a little with your fingers—it should stick together. If it feels too dry, add a little more coconut oil and pulse again. Sprinkle the crumble on top of the berries, making sure to cover them evenly. Add the poppy seeds on top for extra crunch.

Bake for 20 to 30 minutes, or until the crumble top is golden and the berries have softened to release some juices. Remove the crumble from the oven, let it cool for a few minutes, and serve each portion with a dollop of chamomile and lavender coconut cream.

recipe continues on page 176

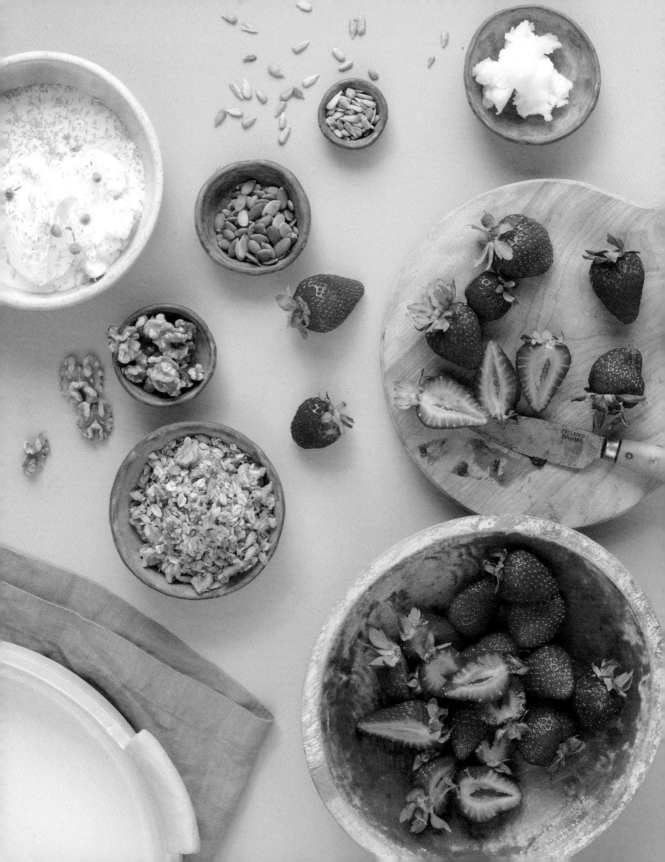

Chamomile and Lavender Coconut Cream

MAKES ABOUT 1 CUP

One 13.5-ounce can full-fat
coconut milk

1 tablespoon chamomile
flowers, dried

½ teaspoon lavender, dried

½ teaspoon vanilla extract

½ tablespoon maple syrup, or liquid
sweetener of choice

Edible flowers (page 70), for garnish

A day before making your crumble, open the can of coconut milk and pour into a bowl. Whisk and add in the chamomile and lavender. Allow the mixture to sit overnight on the counter. In the morning, strain out the herbs, and then add to a jar to store in the fridge until it's solid. This should take about 2 hours to set.

When the crumble is just about done, remove the jar from the fridge and scoop out the thick layer of solid cream and place into a bowl. Store the remaining coconut liquid in a jar for later use. Whisk the cream gently with a fork, adding vanilla and maple syrup, and dollop onto the warm crumble just before serving. Garnish the dessert with fresh or dried chamomile, lavender, and/or crushed rose petals. Store extra in the fridge for up to 3 days. ∎

Raw Reishi Mousse Cups with Cardamom Coconut Cream

Our go-to medicinal mushroom is the prized *Ganoderma lucidum*, or reishi. Known as the "mushroom of immortality," reishi has been revered for centuries in China and Japan for its ability to support the circulatory, respiratory, nervous, immune, and digestive systems. It's a wonderful ally against stress and the toxic load of modern times.

Dark chocolate and reishi are a match made in heaven. This simple mousse is a rich dessert that's not overly sweet. The chocolate and tahini are a great complement to the earthy medicinal mushrooms, and a dollop of fresh cardamom coconut cream helps balance the richness. We recommend, like all summer desserts, serving with a sprinkle of edible flowers for an extra-special treat. MAKES 4 MOUSSE CUPS

Scant one 13.5-ounce can (1 cup) full-fat coconut milk

½ tablespoon reishi powder

1¼ cup bittersweet chocolate, chopped

⅔ cup tahini or sunflower butter

Pinch of sea salt

2 to 4 tablespoons maple syrup, to taste

Flaky sea salt, to garnish

FOR THE CARDAMOM COCONUT CREAM

One 13.5-ounce can full-fat coconut milk, kept cold in the fridge

½ teaspoon ground cardamom

Edible flowers (page 70), optional

In a small saucepan over low heat, warm the 1 cup of coconut milk just enough to steam but not to boil. While the milk is warming, combine the reishi powder, chocolate, tahini, and salt in a mixing bowl. Pour the warm milk over the mixture and stir with a wooden spoon until the chocolate is melted and smooth. Then add 1 tablespoon of maple syrup at a time, tasting until it's sweet enough for your liking. Pour the mousse evenly among four shallow cups and sprinkle each with flaky sea salt before popping them in the fridge to set for about 2 hours.

Now for the cardamom coconut cream. This can be made ahead with the mousse or whipped up just before serving. Simply scoop out the cream, about 1 cup, from the top of a can of cold coconut milk into a small mixing bowl and reserve the rest for another use. Sprinkle in the cardamom and stir with a spoon to combine. Add a dollop of the cardamom coconut cream to the mousse cups just before serving. Top with edible flowers for an extra-special dessert. ▪

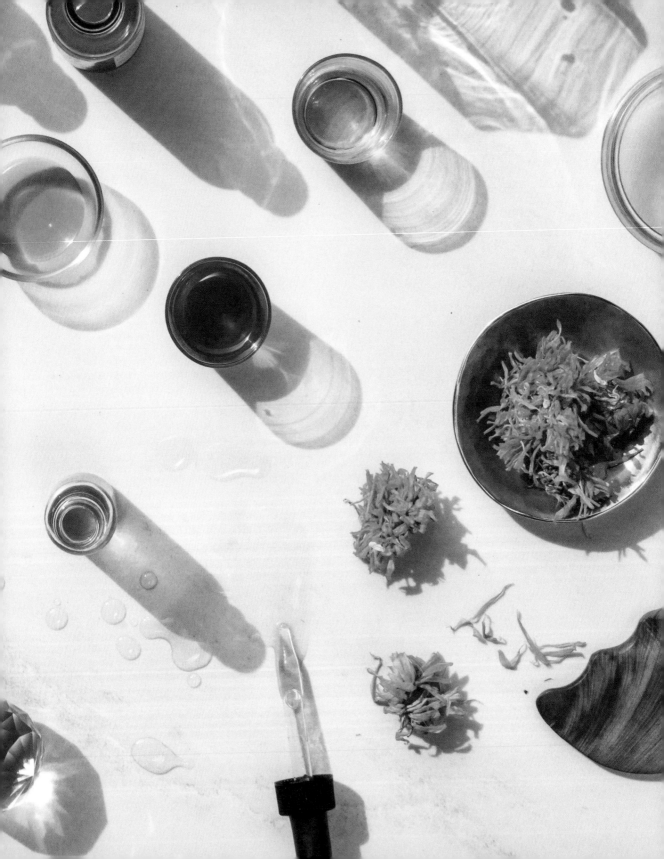

Summer Rituals for Transformation

During this expansive time of year, we're finally ready to bloom. We're doing, being, and expanding into our purpose, and it can be easy to overdo it and get overheated. Though our days may be busy and invigorating, it's important to take a siesta in the afternoon so the body can integrate all this fresh new energy.

We like to focus on cooling and restorative practices to help us bring all this warm and active energy of summer into balance. This could look like a daily sun meditation, yin yoga, massage for overworked muscles or abhyanga with cooling oils. Whatever you do, just remember to set aside time to take it easy and soak up the glow of summer.

MORNING MEDITATION

When you wake up with the sun, everything feels brighter. Try creating a morning meditation routine practiced outside in the sunshine and open air. To start, simply breathe in deeply and count how long it takes to fully expand your lungs. Then, on the out-breath, release the air, taking twice as long as you did on the in-breath. This will deeply reset and relax your parasympathetic nervous system. After doing this exercise for 1 to 2 minutes, resume normal breathing. Focus on your breath, and while thoughts might come up, there's no need to worry or focus on anything specific. Just let your thoughts pass and focus on the breath and the feeling of the warm light of the sun. Call in calm and abundance. You can set a timer if you like; we suggest doing a 20-minute grounding meditation each day—but even just 5 minutes can be life changing over time.

COOL OFF WITH SOOTHING HERBS AND OILS

With the long and bright days of summer, the end of the day can leave you feeling burned out—in more ways than one! By pairing cooling rituals and herbs with the season, we can create more balance. We like to use coconut oil or a Cooling Infused Herbal Oil (page 180) in our seasonal massage rituals. Massage into the body with long gliding strokes towards the heart or the soles of your feet before tucking in after a long sunny day.

Another way to bring down the heat is with a cold herbal compress. Simply make a tea with your favorite cooling skin-nourishing herbs, like chamomile and lavender, and then allow the tea to cool. Soak a washcloth in the tea, and apply to the forehead, neck, chest, or feet. This is especially restorative after a hike or a long day of gardening.

Cooling Infused Herbal Oils

It's easy to get overheated, dry, and inflamed during the hotter months. Nourishing and protecting your skin with cooling oils will help prevent and treat seasonal irritations. Some of the best oils for summer are inexpensive and probably already in your pantry. Coconut, hemp, and sunflower oil are lighter weight and easily absorb into the skin. It can be nice to apply cooling oils to the body after a shower. Use enough oil so you feel moisturized but not so much that the oil doesn't sink in after a few minutes. Apply the oil starting at your feet, working your way to your upper body.

To get even more benefit from cooling oils, try infusing them with cooling herbs. Making a medicated oil is inexpensive and easier than you think! It also ensures you're getting the purest oil with no additives. Working with dried plants and herbs is a great introduction to making infused oils. See our favorite herbs to use on page 180. By using dried plants, you're less likely to have moisture get into the oil, which can cause it to go rancid. Herbal-infused oils are great to have on hand to use on their own or as the base for salves and other topical preparations. FILLS 1 QUART-SIZED JAR

Dried herbs (see next page)   **Oil of your choice, such as coconut (melted), sunflower, hemp, or olive**

Fill your clean and dry quart-sized mason jar halfway with dried herbs—either a single herb or a blend. Pour the oil over the herbs and use a chopstick or wooden spoon to mix, making sure the herbs are completely covered and saturated. Close the jar with a tight-fitting lid and add a label with the plants used, type of oil, and date. Store in a cool place for 3 to 6 weeks, making sure to shake the jar at least once a week.

When your infused oil is ready, strain out the herbs. Line a metal strainer with cheesecloth and place over a mixing bowl. Pour the jar of herbs into the strainer, gathering the edges of the cheesecloth so you can wring out as much of the oil as possible. Pour the oil into a clean mason jar with a tight-fitting lid. Infused oils will keep for about 1 year if stored in a cool place. ∎

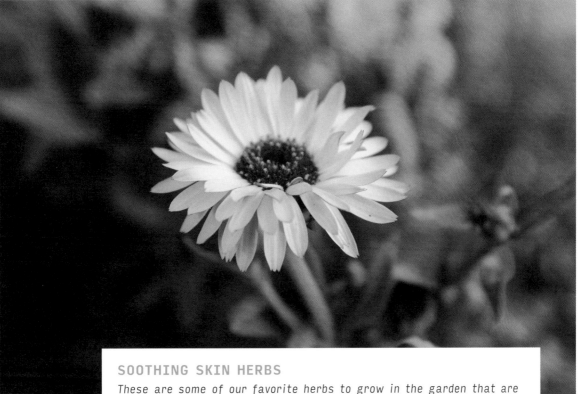

SOOTHING SKIN HERBS

These are some of our favorite herbs to grow in the garden that are allies both internally and externally. Save some to dry and use for making herbal oils to soothe inflamed skin, cuts, and bruises. They are also easy to find dried; see our resources section (page 249).

CALENDULA: This plant, with its bright cheerful blooms, is one of the best herbs for the skin. Calendula is a gentle healer that can have powerful results soothing dry or irritated skin and healing cuts and burns. Its anti-inflammatory and antiseptic properties make it a wonderful ally when spending more time outdoors. Calendula oil has a pleasant slightly floral smell and a rich golden hue.

LAVENDER: Just the familiar scent of lavender flowers is instantly soothing. Lavender helps calm inflamed skin and heal bites, bruises, and burns. It can also help relax tight muscles, which often occur for those who run hot.

PLANTAIN: If you're not familiar with plantain, you'll be surprised to know that it's likely already growing in the neglected areas of your yard or garden. Broadleaf plantain, Plantago major, has ribbed tongue-shaped leaves with tall and slender flower spikes that make them easy to spot. If you ever get a bite or sting, a direct application of plantain will help relieve the inflammation and lessen the pain. As a daily oil, plantain will help calm and moisturize dry, irritated skin.

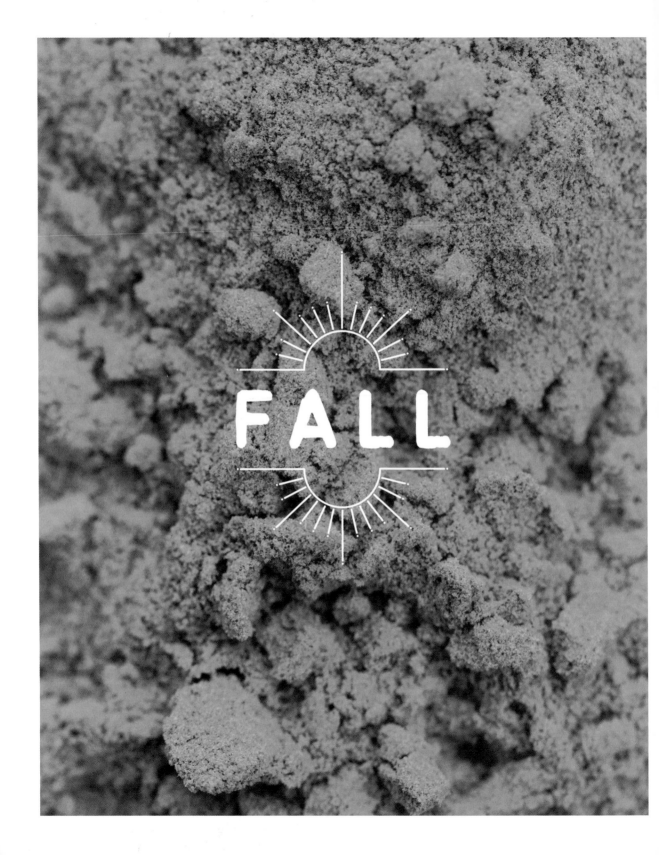

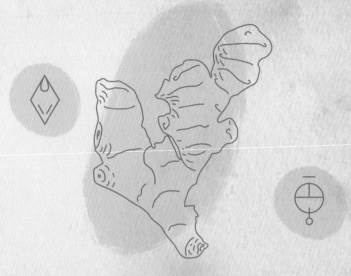

FALL INVITES US TO GATHER THE FRUITS WE PLANTED DURING the summer months. This is a time when we begin to reseed and prepare for the cold days ahead. We can feel the change in our environment in the crispness of the air. Trees shed the last of their leaves and the earth prepares to go inward by drying up, beckoning the green plant beings to rest in her rich soils.

This time of year is synonymous with the elements of vata, reminding us to nourish and ground ourselves. To ward off cold and dry imbalances, it's important to focus on foods that have the opposite qualities: heavy, oily, and moistening. Look for flavors that are wholesomely sweet such as root vegetables, squash, and pumpkins. Soups and stews are perfect for daily meals, as they provide easily digestible nutrients that keep skin, hair, and nails supple. Enjoying seaweeds cooked in broths and adding sea salt to meals will help moisten the body as well. It's no surprise that many foods during this time of year feature warming herbs and spices—apples stewed in cinnamon, squash with savory garlic and sage, a warm mug of tea sprinkled with nutmeg—these flavors impart comfort and nostalgia as well as aid in warming the body and stoking digestive fire.

As the season is changing, rituals should transition from the lighter cooling qualities of summer to heavier warming qualities. Taking hot baths to soothe muscles and calm any anxiety will be a key practice to balance vata in the body. Slathering on and massaging skin with oils will help create a protective barrier from the dry air and further relax the nervous system. Taking time to give extra attention to the body through food, herbs, and rituals will make you less susceptible to the common colds floating around this time of year. Spending time listening to your body, making space to be alone, and enjoying the stillness of resting are just what this season calls for.

FOODS	HERBS	RITUALS	REDUCE
Wet and hydrating cooked foods, such as soups, stews, and broths	Grounding and warming spices: cardamom, cayenne, cinnamon, ginger, lemongrass, rosemary, sage, thyme	Warming Winter Salt Scrub (page 244)	Bitter, astringent, cold, and raw foods
Grounding starchy vegetables and roots such as beets, carrots, squash, sweet potatoes, and turnips	Nutritive nervous system herbs: chamomile, lavender, milky oats, passionflower, skullcap	Warm, hydrating herbal baths and Herbal Steams (page 146)	Pickled foods, ferments, vinegars
Broths and salted water for hydration with added electrolytes	Warming and building adaptogens: ashwagandha, eleuthero, licorice, maca	Daily Abhyanga (page 214) with warming oils, such as sesame and oil infused with ashwagandha	Crunchy and dry foods and snacks
Supplement with healthy fats and essential fatty acids, such as evening primrose, ghee, and olive oil, to balance the dryness of the season		Swabbing sesame oil in the nose and ears to soothe dry skin	Ice cream and cold drinks
		Grounding breath work	Caffeine
		Light exercise and movement that focuses on flow, such as restorative yoga and swimming	Exposure to cold and wind
			Time spent on technology
			Impromptu travel and decision-making

FALL SEASON

ELEMENTS: Ether and air

QUALITIES: Cold and dry

DOSHA: Vata

BALANCING FALL FLAVORS: Sweet, salty, sour, spicy, pungent

SIGNALS OF BALANCE: Feeling grounded and embodied, having a sense of calm and trust, creating nourishing routines, eating consistently, glowing, hydrated, vibrant

SIGNALS OF IMBALANCE: Feeling cold, dry skin and hair, easily irritated, having a lack of focus, depleted nervous system, fatigue, easily overwhelmed, anxious or fearful, tendency toward constipation, dehydration

Everyday Fall Brew

Winds of change call for grounded, rooted energy. That's why we lean into nervines and warming spices for the cool fall season. While fall can represent change and transition, it's also a time to celebrate our final harvest—both literally and figuratively.

As with any transition, this cooler season can bring up anxiety and exacerbate dryness. This is why we need to focus on soothing and nourishing plants such as fennel and marshmallow root, which support the digestive system and soothe internal tissues. We've also added in skullcap, which is a nervine that works both acutely and over time to restore proper nervous system function. The cold and dry qualities can easily create anxiety and stress when they're in excess, so it's important to rely on grounding practices and calming herbs during this season. FILLS 1 PINT-SIZED JAR

1 cup dried skullcap

2½ tablespoons dried fennel seed

2½ tablespoons dried cinnamon chips

2 tablespoons dried marshmallow root, optional

+ NOTE: All herbs should be cut and sifted

Mix the herbs and spices in a bowl to combine and pour the mixture into a labeled pint-sized jar. Store in a cool, dark place.

To make a daily quart of tea, add 2 to 3 tablespoons (about 1 teaspoon or more per cup) of the blend to a muslin bag or tea pouch and place inside a quart-sized mason jar. Preheat the jar with warm water on the outside, then fill with hot water for tea. Cover and allow the mixture to infuse for about 15 to 20 minutes; use the Hot Water Herbal Infusion method (page 94) as inspiration. Take out the herbs and enjoy this fall brew throughout the day, adding honey or lemon to taste. We suggest sipping on about 2 to 4 cups throughout the day to get the most benefit. You can store the tea in the fridge for up to 2 days. ■

Ashwagandha Turmeric Golden Milk Elixir

Not only does adding herbs such as turmeric or ashwagandha to milk have a delicious flavor, but it also has a medicinal action in its own right by maximizing the grounding and moistening properties of the herbs. This elixir leans on turmeric's properties to promote healthy digestion and support healthy liver function. And with the addition of ashwagandha, it helps promote restful sleep. It's a wonderful remedy to enjoy before bed, helping you digest, unwind, and ground into your body.

MAKES 1 CUP

¼ to ½ teaspoon ashwagandha powder

¼ teaspoon ground turmeric

⅛ teaspoon ground cardamom

1 cup milk, we recommend full-fat coconut milk from a can or homemade nut milk (page 90)

1 teaspoon Ghee (page 110) or coconut oil

Maple syrup or stevia to taste, optional

In a saucepan over medium-low heat, add the ashwagandha, turmeric, and cardamom and whisk in the milk. Bring to a simmer for 5 minutes, then remove from the heat. Stir in the ghee. Add the sweetener, if using. Pour the milk into a mug and dust the top with a pinch of ground cardamom. ∎

HALDI DOODH

Haldi doodh, or turmeric milk, is a traditional drink served throughout India as a remedy for everything from digestive issues to muscle soreness and pain. While this rhizome has recently gained a cult following in the wellness world and beyond for its anti-inflammatory properties, turmeric has been used medicinally since ancient times in Ayurvedic, Chinese, and Unani medicine for its affinity to soothe mucous membranes, encourage appetite, and reduce gas and bloating.

Adaptogenic Luna Chai Concentrate

This twist on chai combines many of our favorite herbal allies for supporting moon-time balance. The key herb in this blend is vitex (*Vitex agnus-castus*), which is used in Western herbalism to balance hormones by supporting the pituitary gland—a major player in our endocrine system. There's also dandelion root to support the liver, which is often taxed when we experience the cold quality and general stagnation, which can cause irregularity and cramping during menstrual cycles. Our livers also process and break down excess hormones, so dandelion root helps us have clearer skin.

Stress is also a major player when it comes to hormone imbalance, and it can easily affect us during the vata season. We suggest using maca or ashwagandha as your adaptogens in this blend, as their warming qualities remedy the often cold and constricted energy of the fall. FILLS 1 QUART-SIZED JAR, SERVES 8

5 cups water

2 cinnamon sticks

4-inch thumb fresh ginger, chopped

½ teaspoon whole cloves

1 tablespoon cardamom pods

3 whole star anise

1 tablespoon adaptogenic powder of choice or cut and sifted herb, optional

2 teaspoons dried, cut and sifted roasted dandelion root

2 teaspoons dried vitex berries

4 rooibos tea bags

½ tablespoon vanilla extract

3 tablespoons raw local honey or sweetener of choice

Bring the water to a boil in a large pot, then reduce to a steady simmer. Add in everything except the honey. Allow the herb and spice mixture to simmer, covered, on low (decoct) for about 20 minutes. The water should reduce to about 4 cups.

Turn off the heat and allow the concentrate to sit and cool for another 5 to 10 minutes. Once the concentrate has cooled down a bit, strain out the herbs using a mesh strainer with cheesecloth or a coffee filter. Stir in the honey while warm so that it all dissolves but isn't cooked.

We suggest pouring the concentrate into a prewarmed quart-sized mason jar for storage. It's important that the glass is warm before pouring; if it's cold, the heat of the concentrate will break the jar. Allow the jar to sit out and reach room temperature before storing in your fridge for the week.

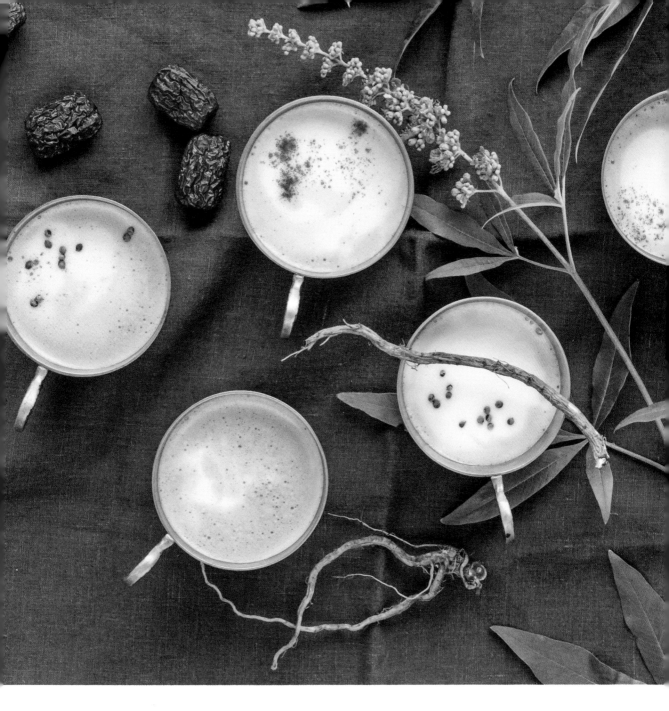

The more honey you add, the longer it will stay preserved. We suggest drinking within 4 days. But this chai is so good, we doubt it will last you more than a few days. It's best to have 2 to 3 cups a day to achieve the medicinal benefits. You can always triple this recipe on your prep day to make sure you have enough.

Serve the beverage hot: 1 part milk of choice to 1 part luna chai concentrate. ■

Spiced Mulled Wine with Hawthorn Berries

A cool weather classic that gets an herbal upgrade, this mulled wine will surely bring warmth and relaxation to your evening. Bright red hawthorn berries can be harvested in fall and early winter and dried to use for months to come. Medicinally, the berries act as a heart tonic, helping normalize blood pressure, strengthen blood flow to the heart, and maintain healthy cholesterol levels. The folklore and magic of this ancient tree has a long history across many cultures. Branches were used for decoration during marriage ceremonies to impart blessings and prosperity.

Energetically, hawthorn is attuned to the heart, helping ease heartache and emotional wounds, which makes this drink a wonderful ally when heading into the colder, darker months of the year. FILLS 1 QUART-SIZED JAR

1 bottle (750 ml) red wine

1/4 cup brandy or whiskey

1/2 cup dried hawthorn berries

2 sweet apples, cored and diced

1/2 tablespoon cardamom pods

4 whole star anise

2 cinnamon sticks, plus more to serve

1/4 cup raw local honey, optional

Add all the ingredients, except the honey, to a medium-sized saucepan and bring to a boil. Turn the heat to low and simmer for 15 to 20 minutes, letting the flavors infuse and the apples soften and release their juice. Scoop out the hawthorn berries, apples, and spices with a small mesh strainer or slotted spoon. Remove from heat and stir in honey, adding more to taste. Serve the mulled wine in mugs, each with a cinnamon stick. Any leftover wine can be refrigerated in a tightly sealed mason jar for about 1 week. ■

Tom Kha Gai with Rice Noodles with Lemon Balm

This flavorful, creamy, and warming soup is perfect for cold and windy fall days. It's building, warming, calming, and it has the perfect balance of sweet, spicy, and restorative—everything you need. As a nervine, lemon balm helps calm the body and mind acutely and more deeply when used consistently over time. Herbalists call it "the bringer of gladness," as it's uplifting and holds a powerful, bright energy. It's also great for calming a nervous stomach suffering from indigestion.

SERVES 4 TO 5

Two 13.5-ounce cans full-fat coconut milk

4 cups chicken or vegetable broth

4 makrut lime leaves

2 stalks lemongrass, sliced

3-inch thumb fresh ginger, sliced

2 tablespoons dried, cut and sifted lemon balm, or 1 small bunch fresh lemon balm

2 cups fresh shiitake mushrooms, chopped; optional

2 to 3 tablespoons fish sauce

2 tablespoons coconut or brown sugar

Juice of 2 limes

1 teaspoon sea salt

8 ounces rice noodles

½ cup freshly chopped lemon balm and/or cilantro, for garnish

Chili oil

1 lime, sliced for garnish

To a heavy-bottomed soup or clay pot, add the coconut milk, broth, makrut lime leaves, lemongrass, ginger, and lemon balm. You can add these herbs to a muslin bag to make them easier to fish out later. Bring the mixture to a simmer and allow the soup to cook on low to medium heat for 15 to 20 minutes. Strain out the herbs, then add the soup back to the pot along with shiitake mushrooms, fish sauce, and sugar to cook on low for 10 minutes. Then add in the juice of two limes and salt to taste.

While the broth is simmering, prep the rice noodles according to the instructions on the package. They should take just 5 minutes to boil in water, then strain and leave in cool water until the noodles are ready to serve.

Divide the broth between serving bowls and add in the noodles. Top with fresh herbs such as lemon balm or cilantro, drizzle with chili oil, and serve with lime slices on the side. You can also add in shredded chicken or diced tofu for some extra protein. This dish is fun to mix up with all sorts of veggies, such as shredded cabbage, thinly sliced peppers, and julienned carrots—the more the merrier. ■

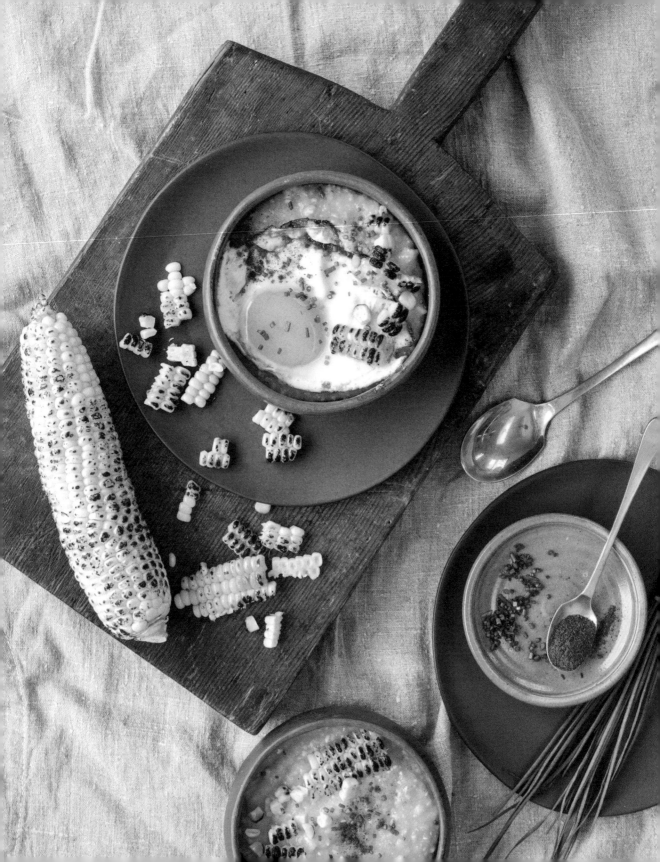

Bone Broth Breakfast Grits

Grits are a southern comfort food we ate growing up in Florida, enjoying a hot bowl—with lots of butter and scrambled eggs mixed in—for breakfast on school days. There's something so satisfying about simple dishes like grits.

This recipe is a slightly elevated version of our childhood "grits 'n' eggs" days. The addition of mineral-rich, gut-healing bone broth helps offset the drying qualities of the corn, imparts a deeper flavor, and infuses medicinal herbs into the meal. Adding in dried roots that support the immune system, such as astragalus, gives extra support to your immune system before cold and flu season hits. The runny yolks of the eggs are high in lecithin, a protein that nourishes the nervous system by supporting the myelin sheath that surrounds the nerve endings. **SERVES 2**

4 cups Everyday Herbal Bone Broth (page 112)

2 teaspoons sea salt

¼ teaspoon smoked paprika

2 cups stone-ground cornmeal grits or polenta

2 teaspoons Ghee (page 110), plus more for serving

2 eggs

Chives, chopped for garnish

Olive oil, optional

Fresh cracked black pepper, optional

In a medium saucepan, bring the bone broth to a boil. Season with sea salt and smoked paprika, then begin whisking as you add in the grits to prevent clumping. Turn down to a simmer, stirring the grits every few minutes until the cornmeal is soft and the texture is creamy, about 20 minutes. Add more liquid to thin out the grits if needed.

When the grits are just about done, cook your eggs. Add 2 teaspoons of ghee to a cast-iron skillet and melt on medium heat. When pan is hot, crack in both eggs, cooking until their edges are slightly brown and crispy. Turn off the heat and carefully flip over the eggs to just barely set the yolk. You want the yolks to remain runny, so only leave them in the skillet for about 30 seconds. To serve, spoon a cup or so of grits into two bowls with a dollop of ghee, then top each with an egg. Garnish with an extra pinch of smoked paprika and a sprinkle of chopped chives. Add a drizzle of good olive oil and fresh cracked black pepper, if you like. Keep any extra grits for leftovers or for breakfast the following day. ■

Pumpkin Apple Kosmic Kurry Soup

Making curries in the fall encourages warmth in our bodies and digestive systems. Crafting your own spice blend is a great way to play up the flavors you love and incorporate more healing adaptogens into everyday meals. This curry uses red kuri, a Japanese squash with a sweet, rich taste and a thin skin, so there's no need to peel it before eating or cooking. Look for red kuri squash in natural food stores or at your local farmers market and stock up, since they will last throughout the winter. SERVES 6 TO 8

1 small red kuri squash or butternut squash

½ tablespoon olive oil, to rub on the squash skin plus more for garnish

1 tablespoon Ghee (page 110), or coconut oil

1 onion, diced

1 tablespoon Kosmic Kurry Spice Blend (page 99)

1 russet or red potato, diced with skin on

1-inch thumb fresh ginger, minced

2 apples, cored and diced

1 cinnamon stick

4 cups Everyday Herbal Bone Broth (page 112), veggie broth, or water

1 tablespoon white miso paste

1 teaspoon sea salt, optional

Full-fat plain yogurt, for garnish

Fresh cilantro, for garnish

Preheat the oven to 350°F. Cut the squash in half and brush the skin with olive oil, placing it cut side down on a parchment-lined baking sheet. Bake for about 30 minutes or until tender and easily pierced with a fork.

While the squash is roasting, add ghee or coconut oil to a heavy-bottomed soup pot and melt on medium heat. Add in the onion and let soften, cooking for about 5 minutes. Next, add in the Kosmic Kurry Spice Blend, stirring to coat the onion. Add in the potato, ginger, apples, and cinnamon stick, stirring well. Pour in the broth and increase the heat to bring the soup to a simmer.

Once the squash is cooked, let it cool for a few minutes and then carefully scoop out the seeds and remove the stem. Break or cut the squash into large pieces and add it to the soup pot, skin and all. If using butternut, don't include the skin, as it can be tough. Let the soup simmer for 20 to 30 minutes, then turn off the heat.

Thin the miso paste by adding it to a small bowl and pouring over a few splashes of hot (not boiling) water and whisk until smooth. This will prevent the miso from becoming lumpy in the soup. Add the thinned miso paste into the soup

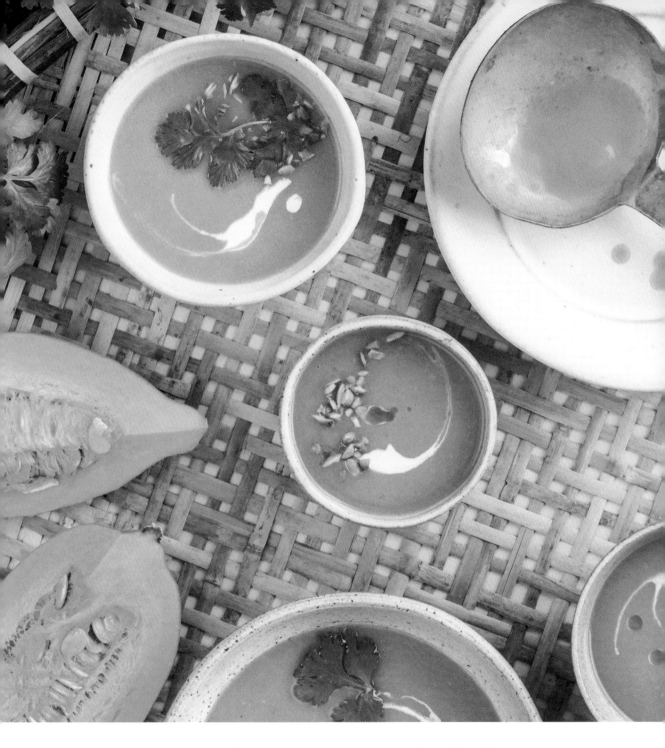

and stir to combine. Remove the cinnamon stick and blend the soup to a creamy consistency with a hand blender or in batches in a high-speed blender. Season with sea salt if needed and stir well. To serve, divide among bowls and add a dollop of plain yogurt, a drizzle of olive oil, and a few cilantro leaves. ■

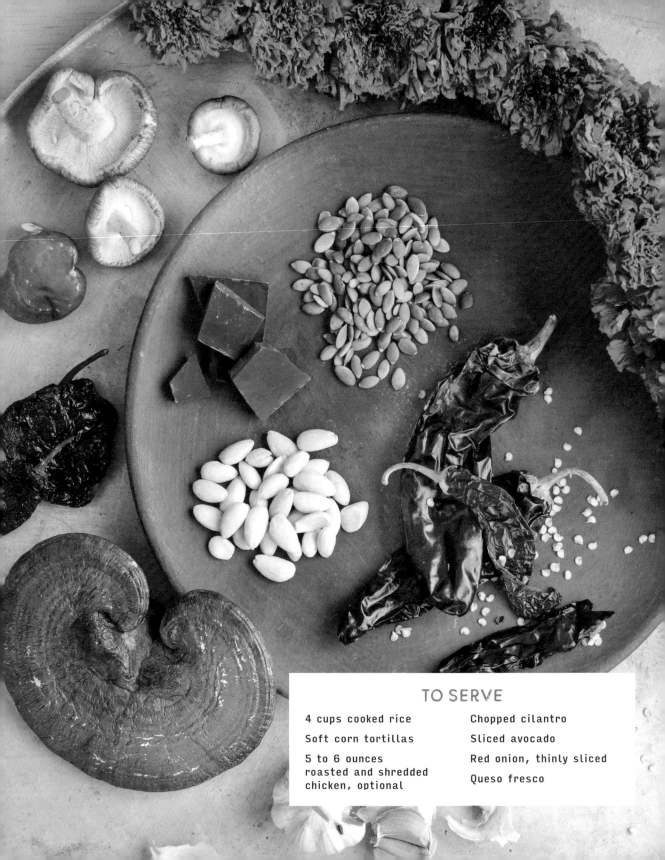

TO SERVE

4 cups cooked rice

Soft corn tortillas

5 to 6 ounces
roasted and shredded
chicken, optional

Chopped cilantro

Sliced avocado

Red onion, thinly sliced

Queso fresco

Magical Mushroom Mole

OK, so this mole is not truly made with "magic" mushrooms, but the medicinal fungi used are out of this world! Traditional moles are made with all kinds of different ingredients, depending on the chef and the region in which it's made. We enjoyed so many different flavors and styles of mole during our time in Oaxaca, Mexico, where some of the original moles come from.

The word *mole* simply means "sauce." In Mexico you'll find mole that's red, green, brown, and in other varieties and textures. Here in the United States we usually find the dark brown mole, which is infused with peppers and dark chocolate. It's the perfect combination of sweet and savory flavors and happens to be an ideal vehicle for medicinal mushrooms. SERVES 4 TO 5

5 pasilla and/or ancho chilis, chopped and deseeded

2 tablespoons coconut oil or Ghee (page 110)

1 yellow onion, chopped

2 cloves garlic, chopped

1 teaspoon ground cinnamon

1 teaspoon ground cumin

1 teaspoon ground coriander

2 cups chicken or vegetable broth

5 ounces Oaxacan or dark chocolate

¼ cup chopped, blanched, and toasted almonds

¼ cup toasted pumpkin seeds

¼ cup raisins

1 teaspoon dried oregano

1 tablespoon brown or coconut sugar, optional

1 to 1½ tablespoons powdered reishi mushrooms, and/or chaga, shiitake, and maitake

Sea salt to taste

Soak the chilies in about 1 cup of water for 15 to 20 minutes. While soaking, add coconut oil to a medium saucepan on low to medium heat, add in the onion, and sauté until translucent. Then add in the garlic, cinnamon, cumin, and coriander to release their flavors. This should take 5 to 10 minutes.

Next, strain your soaked chilies and discard the water. Pour the chilies and the onion mixture into a blender or food processor along with the broth, chocolate, almonds, pumpkin seeds, raisins, oregano, sugar, and mushroom powder. Blend until super smooth, then return to the saucepan and bring the sauce to a simmer. Cook the mole on low for 20 to 25 minutes.

Serve over or alongside the cooked rice. Or toss the chicken in the sauce and wrap in warm corn tortillas. Garnish with chopped cilantro, sliced avocado, thinly sliced red onions, and queso fresco. ■

Crispy Salmon with Adaptogenic Ginger Maca Miso Sauce and Roasted Radishes with Herb Butter

We're always looking for ways to use our creamy Adaptogenic Ginger Maca Miso Dressing (page 106) and this recipe is no exception. This simple stovetop preparation for salmon is a breeze and leaves the fish moist and tender. Roasting radishes brings out a deeper flavor and softens their spicy kick. Let them get nice and crispy around the edges and tender on the inside. Tossing the radishes in herb butter only makes them better, and you can save any extra butter for other vegetables throughout the week. **SERVES 2**

1 bunch Easter egg radishes or baby turnips, trimmed and sliced lengthwise

½ tablespoon Ghee (page 110), melted

Sea salt

¼ pound unsalted butter, softened at room temperature

1 tablespoon freshly chopped parsley, dill, thyme, or fennel

½ teaspoon flake salt

2 salmon fillets, 4 to 6 ounces each

¼ cup Adaptogenic Ginger Maca Miso Dressing (page 106)

2 teaspoons black sesame seeds, for garnish

Preheat the oven to 400°F. On a baking sheet lined with parchment paper, toss the radishes with the melted ghee and a sprinkle of sea salt. Pop them in the oven to roast for about 20 minutes, until they're tender and beginning to brown. While they're roasting, make the herb butter by mixing the softened butter and freshly chopped herbs of choice in a bowl with a fork until well combined. Sprinkle in the flake salt to taste and set aside.

Prep the salmon by sprinkling sea salt on both sides. Add the salmon to an unheated (not preheated) cast-iron skillet, skin side down. Turn the heat to medium and let the salmon cook for 5 minutes without moving. The salmon will be cooked about halfway up the side of each fillet. Turn off the heat and use a spatula to flip the fillets, letting them cook in the residual heat of the pan for about 1 minute. Move the salmon to a plate to rest before serving.

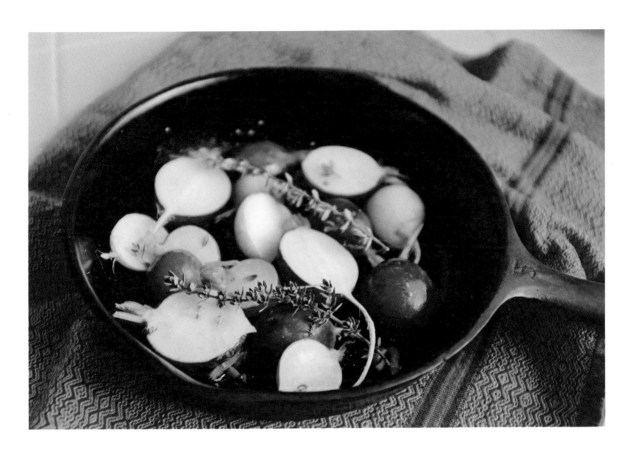

When the radishes are done roasting, remove them from the oven and add 1 tablespoon of herb butter, tossing to make sure they're well coated. To serve, spread a spoonful of Adaptogenic Ginger Maca Miso Dressing onto each plate and place a salmon fillet on top, skin side up. Spoon the herb–buttered radishes onto the plates and add a sprinkle of black sesame seeds on top to garnish. ■

Herby Greek Lemon Soup

We love making this tangy, nutrient-dense citrus soup during fall, as it also happens to be the start of Meyer lemon season here in California. These full, juicy fruits are full of flavor and are a bit sweeter than your average lemon. Our recipe is inspired by a traditional Greek lemon chicken avgolemono, which is a sauce made of egg yolk, lemon, and broth; it's insanely delicious.

We top this soup with whatever seasonal herbs we have handy. In fall, we incorporate fennel, dill, lemon balm, oregano, and parsley. If you're feeling a bit under the weather, you can add in 3 to 4 sticks of astragalus root to keep the seasonal bugs at bay. That combined with the extra garlic in the soup will work to protect and support your immune system as the weather shifts. SERVES 4

2 tablespoons butter, Ghee (page 100), or olive oil

1 small fennel bulb, sliced lengthwise

1 sweet onion, sliced lengthwise

2 garlic cloves, minced

1 bay leaf

4 cups vegetable or chicken broth

2 chicken breasts, optional

Sea salt and black pepper to taste

2 sticks astragalus root, optional

Juice of 3 Meyer (or regular) lemons, plus extra lemon slices for garnish

2 eggs

1 cup cooked orzo

1 cup chopped green seasonal herbs such as parsley, basil, lemon balm, and tulsi; reserve a handful for garnish

Crushed black pepper, for garnish

Olive oil, for garnish

Heat a heavy-bottomed soup pot on low to medium and add in the butter. Next, add in the sliced fennel and onion. Stir and allow the veggies to get mildly translucent, adding in the garlic for the last minute. Add more butter or oil as needed and bring the heat down to low if it begins to simmer. The goal is to smell the aroma of the plants, so their flavors are released into the soup.

Add the bay leaf, broth, and chicken breasts, if using, to the mix. Add a couple of pinches of sea salt, pepper, and astragalus root, if using. Cover and allow the mixture to simmer for about 20 minutes. If added, remove the chicken breast, shred, and return to the broth.

While the soup simmers, whisk together the lemon juice and eggs. After the 20 minutes have passed, add the lemon juice–egg mixture, orzo, and herbs, and cook for a few more minutes before serving. Add more sea salt to taste. The soup will become a beautiful, bright, creamy yellow color. Serve in a bowl with freshly sliced lemons, crushed black pepper, and a sprinkle of fresh herbs. Add a splash of olive oil to each bowl for extra richness and healthy, grounding fatty acids. ■

Escarole Caesar Salad with Seed Cracker Croutons

In the beginning of fall when the days can still be on the warmer side, this escarole version of a Caesar salad is just the thing. Escarole has become one of our favorite bitter greens that is substantial enough to enjoy as a salad on its own or added to brothy soups. It can be difficult to find outside of local farmers markets or specialty foods stores, but it's worth the search. Use radicchio if you can't get your hands on escarole, though it tends to be more bitter. A friend of ours soaks bitter greens in water for a few minutes to help reduce some of the bitterness. Adding nori is a spin-off of the salty anchovies in traditional Caesar dressings. The seed cracker croutons are our version of croutons in this salad, and you can make an extra batch to enjoy throughout the week, as these croutons are excellent on soups, grains, and greens. SERVES 2 TO 4

¹/₄ cup tahini

Juice of 1 lemon

2 garlic cloves, microplaned

1 teaspoon Dijon mustard

¹/₈ teaspoon ground turmeric

¹/₄ teaspoon sea salt

¹/₂ teaspoon freshly cracked black pepper, plus more to serve

2 teaspoons nutritional yeast, optional

3 tablespoons olive oil

1 tablespoon capers, plus more to serve

1 head escarole

1 sheet toasted nori, crumbled

1 cup Seed Crackers (see page 236), broken into crouton-sized pieces

Make the dressing by combining the tahini, lemon juice, garlic, mustard, turmeric, salt, black pepper, and nutritional yeast in a bowl, whisking to combine. Drizzle in the olive oil slowly, whisking until the dressing becomes creamy and emulsified. You can thin out the dressing to your liking by adding a tablespoon of water at a time. Stir in the capers and set aside.

Prep the escarole by cutting off the bottom to easily separate the leaves. Chop the larger leaves in half horizontally to create more manageable pieces, though they should still be substantial, as this is more of a knife-and-fork kind of salad. Using your hands or tongs, toss the escarole in a bowl with 2 tablespoons of the dressing, adding more depending on how much dressing you like. To serve, divide the escarole between plates and top with the extra capers, crumbled toasted nori, seed cracker croutons, and a few cracks of fresh black pepper. ■

Date and Nut Apple Pie Bites

Nothing says fall like apple pie. And apples are a big deal here in west Sonoma County. The heritage variety Gravenstein has been cultivated here for commercial production since the late 1800s and provides the Bay Area with fresh apples all season long. Instead of baking a pie with sugar and flour, we decided to make snack-sized versions to enjoy all the seasonal spices and sweet apples. Maca has a nutty flavor that plays well with walnuts, and is a warming and energizing adaptogen, great for the cooler fall months. You'll likely want to make a double batch of these for easy snacking throughout the week.

MAKES 12 BITES

2 apples, cored and diced

½ tablespoon maca powder

¼ teaspoon ground cinnamon

¼ teaspoon ground ginger

⅛ teaspoon ground nutmeg

Pinch of ground cloves

1 tablespoon water

Pinch of sea salt

1 cup walnuts, toasted

1 cup dates, pitted and chopped

3 tablespoons raw hemp seeds, divided

In a small heavy-bottomed saucepan, add the diced apples, maca powder, spices, and water. Cover and cook over medium heat to let the apples soften, making sure to stir to prevent burning. Once apples are softened, remove from heat and let cool. Then add the mixture to a food processor along with the walnuts, dates, and 1 tablespoon of hemp seeds, and a pinch of sea salt and pulse until the mixture becomes doughlike. Add 1 teaspoon of water at a time if the mixture is too thick and hard to work with. Scrape down the food processor, removing the mixture and adding it to a mixing bowl. On a small plate, add 2 tablespoons of hemp seeds in an even layer. Wet your hands to make the bites easier to handle, then scoop 1 tablespoon of the dough into your hands and roll it into a little ball. Once all the bites are made, roll one side in the hemp seeds. Serve immediately or store in the fridge for up to 1 week. ■

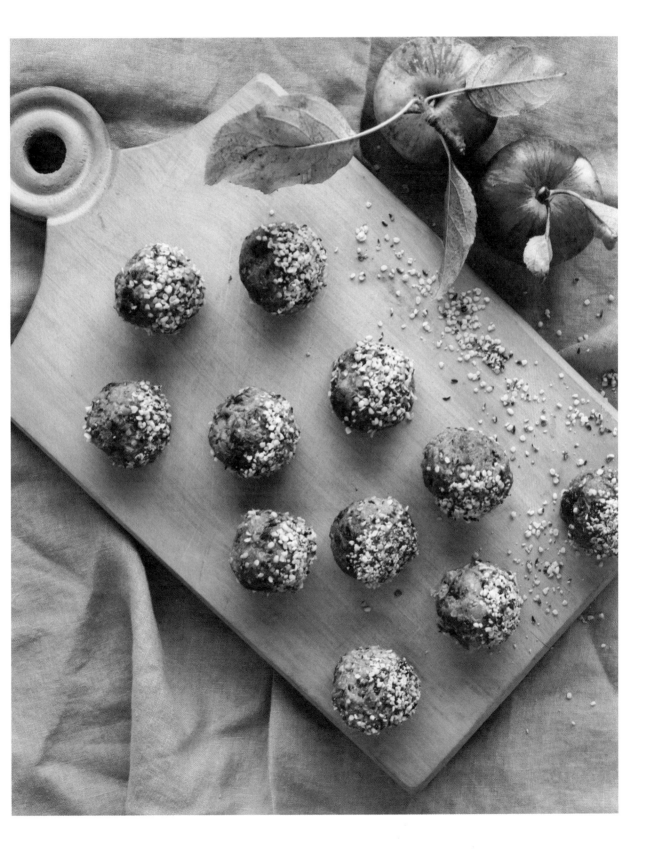

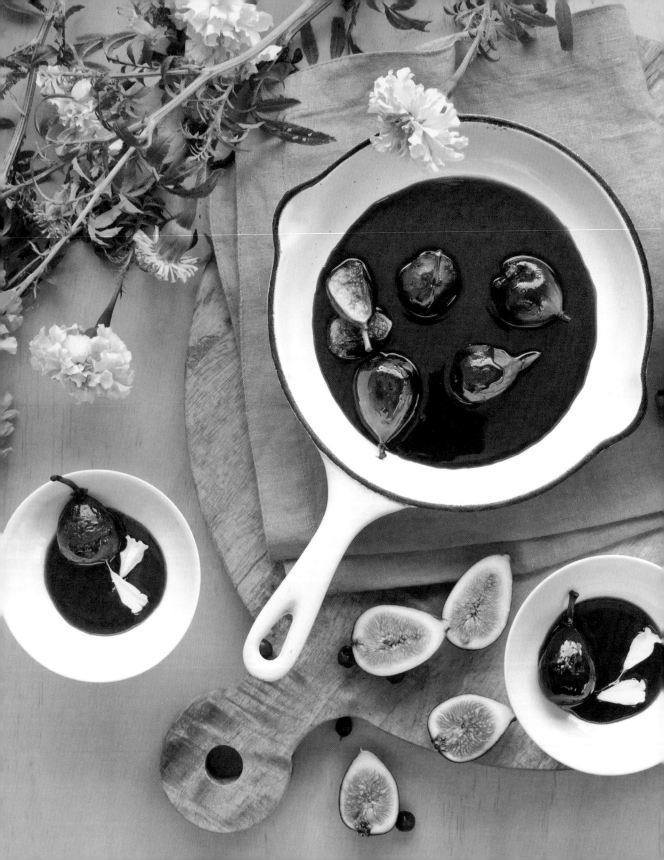

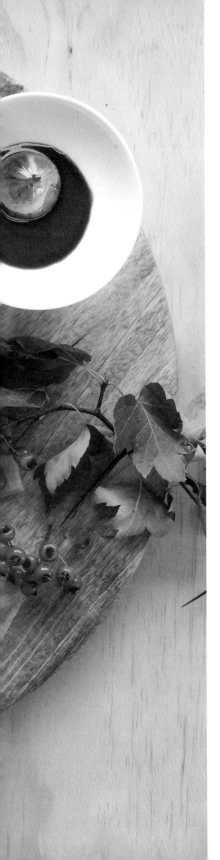

Poached Figs with Spiced Hawthorn Berry Mulled Wine

This is one of those incredibly easy-to-make desserts that looks and tastes decadent. Try to use the freshest figs you can find. Dried figs would work here too, but they'll take a little longer to become soft, so taste first to make sure they're ready before serving. You can make this dairy-free by replacing the crème fraîche with coconut cream. These are fun to serve in little dessert glasses or vintage coupe glasses for an extra-special treat. **SERVES 2**

8 fresh mission figs, stems removed and sliced in half lengthwise

½ cup Spiced Mulled Wine with Hawthorn Berries (page 190 or see note)

¼ cup coconut sugar or maple syrup

3 sprigs fresh thyme

½ cup crème fraîche or coconut cream

+ NOTE: If you don't have any leftover mulled wine, you can make a quick version. Simmer red wine with your favorite spices such as cinnamon, cardamom, or ginger for 10 to 15 minutes.

Add the figs, mulled wine, coconut sugar, and thyme to a saucepan and bring to a boil on medium-high heat. Turn down the heat, reducing the boil to a simmer, and let the wine thicken and reduce to about ¼ cup. Remove from the heat and take out the sprigs of thyme. Divide the crème fraîche between two dessert bowls and top with the figs and syrupy wine. ■

Adaptogenic Power Warming Bites

This is our spin on Rosemary Gladstar's famous "zoom ball" recipe. Rosemary's original recipe calls for stimulating and uplifting herbs, like guarana and kola nut to assist with depleted energy. Our recipes focus on building up a depleted endocrine and nervous system through adaptogens like maca, ashwagandha, and reishi, raising the vibration and health of your entire body.

Changing your behavior and thought patterns and adding in herbs like adaptogens and nervines can help ease the demands of the modern world. We suggest making a batch on your prep day, so you have enough to treat yourself each day and you are consistently getting a dose of herbs. Plus, they are a delicious snack and can make breakfast a breeze.

This recipe is also very adaptable. Add whatever nut butters, powdered herbs, or spices are calling to you—the ones that will help you feel energetically aligned. MAKES 25 ONE-INCH BALLS

One 16-ounce jar nut butter of choice, we like sunflower or cashew

³/₄ cup raw local honey

¹/₂ cup adaptogenic powders

1¹/₂ tablespoons carob powder or unsweetened cocoa powder

¹/₂ teaspoon cinnamon powder

A few pinches of cayenne powder

¹/₂ cup coconut flakes

WARMING ADAPTOGEN OPTIONS

Ashwagandha powder

Astragalus powder

Maca powder

Reishi powder

TOPPINGS

Lightly toasted shredded coconut flakes

Chopped almonds

Toasted sesame seeds

Cocoa powder

Cardamom powder

Cayenne powder

Ginger powder

Crushed rose petals

In a large mixing bowl, combine the nut butter and honey until smooth. Add in the adaptogenic herbal powders you are using, mixing until it all combines. Next, add the carob or cocoa powder, cinnamon, cayenne pepper, and coconut flakes and mix. The consistency should be like a thick paste that is solid enough to roll into balls but not dry enough to feel the powdered herbs. You can add either more powder or nut butter to get the consistency you want.

Wet your hands and roll the dough into silver dollar–sized balls, and then place them on parchment paper or a large plate. Next, create little topping stations with your coconut flakes, cocoa powder, rose petals, sesame seeds, or whatever toppings you choose on small plates. Roll the balls into the toppings to create a beautiful finish. Get creative! Garnish with a pinch of cayenne, or any spice you desire for a little extra flavor. ■

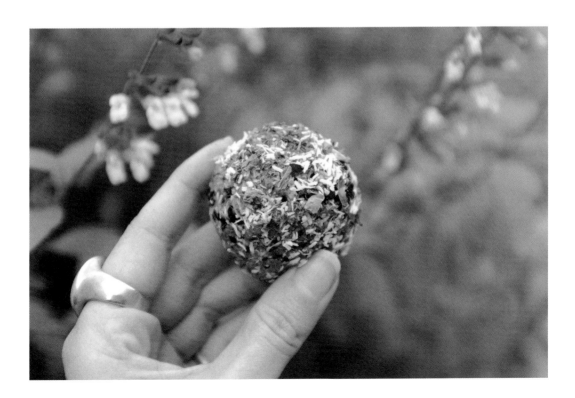

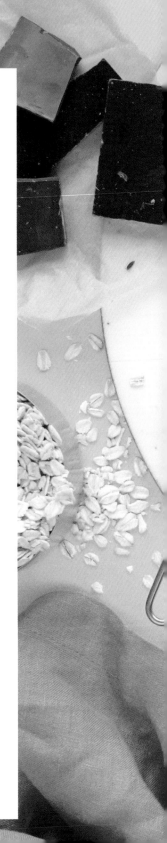

Kosmic Kitchen Sink Cookies with Goji, Maca, and Dark Chocolate

In the heart of fall, it can be hard to resist a good sweet treat. That's why we love prepping a healthy batch of these hearty cookies packed with herbal goodness. They're naturally sweet because of the bananas and coconut oil, and they contain no gluten. We like to use maca root powder, an adaptogen that's easy to find in health food stores with a sweet and nutty taste that's perfect for baking. However, you can also substitute any adaptogenic herbs that are calling to the season or your dosha. MAKES 20 COOKIES

3 large ripe bananas

¼ cup coconut oil, melted

1 teaspoon vanilla extract

3 tablespoons maple syrup

⅔ cup gluten-free flour

2 cups rolled oats

1½ tablespoons maca powder

½ teaspoon of ground cardamom

1 teaspoon ground cinnamon

½ teaspoon sea salt

1 teaspoon baking powder

¼ cup goji berries

¼ cup unsweetened coconut flakes

2 ounces semisweet dark chocolate, chopped

Preheat the oven to 350°F. Peel the bananas and add them to a mixing bowl, mashing them with a fork, whisk, or mixer until smooth. Slowly add in the coconut oil until the mixture becomes a mushy paste. Then mix in the vanilla extract and maple syrup.

Mix the dry ingredients together: the gluten-free flour, oats, maca, cardamom, cinnamon, salt, and baking powder. Then slowly stir the dry ingredients into the bowl with the wet ingredients. Fold in the goji berries, coconut flakes, and the chopped-up semisweet chocolate. You can substitute these "kitchen sink" ingredients for whatever you're craving or what's in season. Once everything is combined, it should have a doughlike consistency.

Line a baking sheet with parchment paper. Wet your hands and form 1-inch-diameter balls from about a spoonful of dough, and then place them on the prepared baking sheet. Bake the cookies for about 20 minutes or until the tops turn a golden hue. Take the cookies out to cool and enjoy. Will last for about 5 days when stored in an airtight container. ■

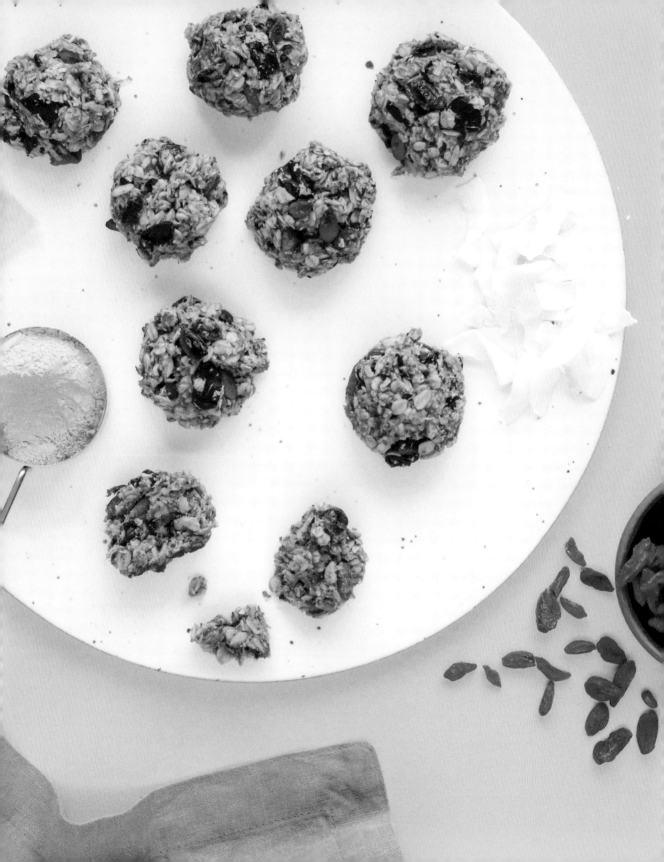

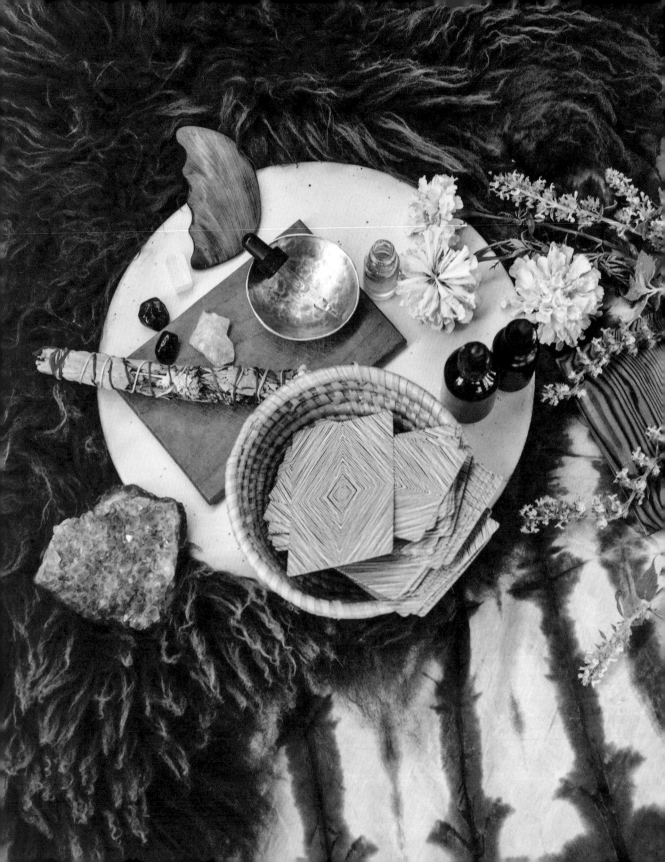

Fall Rituals for Grounding

The fall season is a time to give thanks to the land and ourselves. It's time to celebrate the year's bounty and the beginning of a time of inward growth. In Ayurvedic medicine, fall represents the cold and dry season. In Chinese medicine, it's the end of the yang seasons and the start of the yin cycle, meaning it's a time when we need more nourishment and flow to honor the feminine energy.

Rooted, warming, and hydrating rituals are the name of the game. We like to incorporate more yin yoga, baths, luxurious skin rituals, and general pampering. While summer is a time for high energy with light and bright practices, fall is a time to slow down and reflect. We turn our focus inward, making altars, reflecting on our successes, and getting rooted before the intensity of the dark winter season.

Some of our favorite rituals of the season are decadent and spa-like. Though they can all be prepared at home, if you're pressed for time or just want to, this is the time of year to invest in that facial or try out that body work you've been interested in. We believe self-care rituals are not a luxury but an act of self-preservation to stay in our bodies and the present moment, so we can be our most authentic selves.

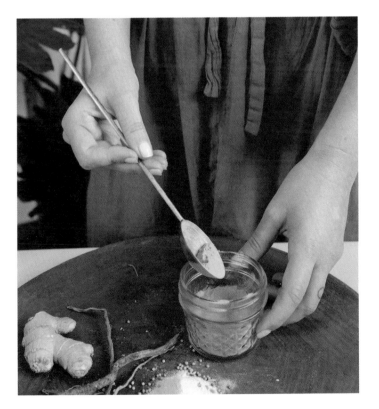

Adaptogenic Honey Face Mask

This mask provides the perfect mix of restoration, hydration, and exfoliation. The honey helps heal any small wounds while also giving the skin a dose of antimicrobial support. The honey and cardamom are both warming and help bring circulation to the surface of the skin. Rose water is toning and tightening and smells divine. We suggest using shatavari root powder during the fall season, as it's moistening and calming. MAKES 1 FACE MASK

1 tablespoon almond flour

½ tablespoon raw local honey

1 teaspoon rose water

1 teaspoon powdered shatavari, or adaptogen of choice

1 pinch ground cardamom

In a small bowl, mix the almond flour and honey together with the rose water. Mix well, then add in the rest of the ingredients and mix until a soft paste is formed. Feel free to tweak the ratios to get a consistency that's to your liking.

Take about a quarter-sized dollop into your palm and use your fingers to gently rub it all over your face. Let the mask sit for 5 to 10 minutes, then rinse it off with warm water. Pat your face dry and follow up with your favorite moisturizer. ■

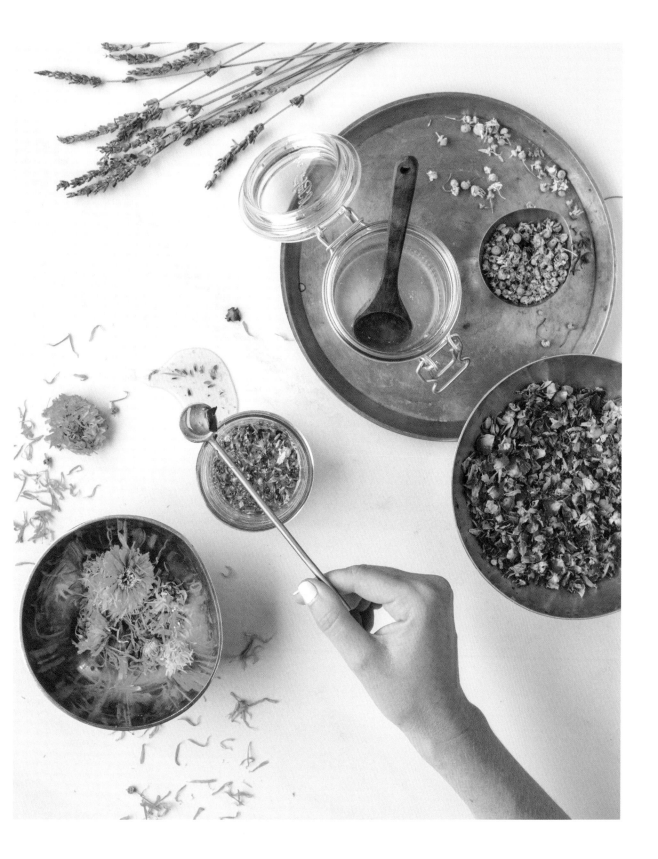

WARMING BODY OILS

You know fall has arrived when you walk outside and it feels like, all of a sudden, there's a crispness in the air and the light has turned a little more golden. The leaves are changing, morphing into a kaleidoscope of bright orange and red hues and drying up as they wait to fall from the trees. That magical shift, as subtle as it can be, lets you know right away that something is different. Our bodies tell us when there's this shift in the seasons. Our skin is the first to notice, often becoming dry from the cooler temperatures and lack of moisture in the air. Since we know fall can be cold and dry, it's important to support our bodies not only from the inside with grounding moistening foods but also from the outside by protecting our skin with warming oils.

This is your cue to switch from the cooling oils you relied on during the hot days of summer to more warming oils that will help insulate you from the cooler days ahead. These oils will be a bit heavier, which will help provide extra nourishment to dry or cracked skin.

SESAME: A slightly nutty oil, sesame is the "king of oils" in Ayurvedic practice. It's warming but not too heavy, and it's easily absorbed by the skin. Sesame oil is often used as the base oil in Ayurvedic medicated oils, which are infused with medicinal herbs to enhance their healing properties.

MAHANARYAN: This deep crimson-colored oil is made with over twenty herbs, including shatavari, ashwagandha, licorice, and ginger, with sesame oil as the base. It's a wonderfully warming oil used to nourish the muscles and joints. The smell isn't quite as neutral as sesame oil due to fragrant herbs such as camphor and neem, though it's pleasant.

ASHWAGANDHA BALA: Strongly scented with warming and strengthening qualities, this oil, which uses sesame oil as the base, is infused with one of our favorite vata-pacifying herbs, ashwagandha. It also includes another warming herb, bala, a member of the mallow family, which gives strength to the body and helps nourish the tissues and calm the nervous system.

CASTOR: Though castor is energetically a cooling oil, it has a unique ability to hold heat when applied warm or when kept warm by using a hot water bottle over the oiled area, such as in castor-oil pack therapies. Castor is deeply nourishing, which is immediately apparent from its thick and heavy texture. Use castor to enhance the richness of lighter oils such as sesame when doing self-massage. On days when your face or lips feel really dry and need extra hydration, add a drop or two in your evening moisturizer before going to bed.

ABHYANGA: SELF-OIL MASSAGE

If you haven't gotten into the practice of self-oil massage, or abhyanga, this is the perfect season to start. When you're feeling dry and cold, you'll be amazed at how soothing this practice is for your skin and nervous system. Abhyanga gives a sense of warmth and comfort not only from the oil sinking into the skin but from the physical act of massaging the body. It's truly a self-nurturing practice that allows you to honor your body and spend time giving gratitude for all that it does.

During the vata season it's easier to experience the elemental imbalances of ether and air. There's a tendency to feel scattered, less grounded, anxious, or fearful emotionally. Doing a self-oil massage helps you come back into your body by putting conscious attention on each part while noticing what the skin, lymph, muscles, and bones feel like. Keeping your oil in a vessel from which it's easy to pour will make the process easier. You can use a glass bottle with a pump or a BPA-free plastic bottle with a pour top, which you'll find many oils already come in.

Here's a simple abhyanga practice to do at home. Try to incorporate this ritual as a daily practice or a few times a week, if you can.

1. Grab your bottle of oil and warm it up by placing it in a jar or mug of hot water for about 5 minutes. You'll need about ¼ cup of oil in the bottle or more.

2. Pour a palmful of the oil into your hands and begin massaging the body, starting at the top of your feet and working your way up toward your head.

3. Massage your limbs using long strokes. When massaging the joints, use circular motions.

4. When you get to your abdomen, massage your belly in a clockwise motion— making a circle starting at the lower right side of the abdomen, ending at the lower left side—so you're following the path of the large intestine.

5. Continue working your way up the body, spending about 10 to 20 minutes total on the massage.

6. If you have the time, rubbing oil into the scalp is deeply relaxing, though not necessary to do every day.

7. Carefully get into a hot bath or shower, making sure to wipe the bottoms of your feet if there's oil on them. Let the warmth of the water open your pores so the oil sinks deeper into the skin. Use soap only where you need to, as you don't want to wash off the oil.

8. When done bathing, pat the body dry with a fresh towel, so as much of the oil stays on the skin as possible.

9. Your skin should feel supple and moisturized, not greasy after drying off. If there's excess oil on the skin, try massaging the oil in deeper next time.

+ SAFETY: Since this is a detoxifying process, it's best to avoid abhyanga during menstruation or pregnancy, or if you have a cold or flu. If you have a medical condition, check with your health-care practitioner.

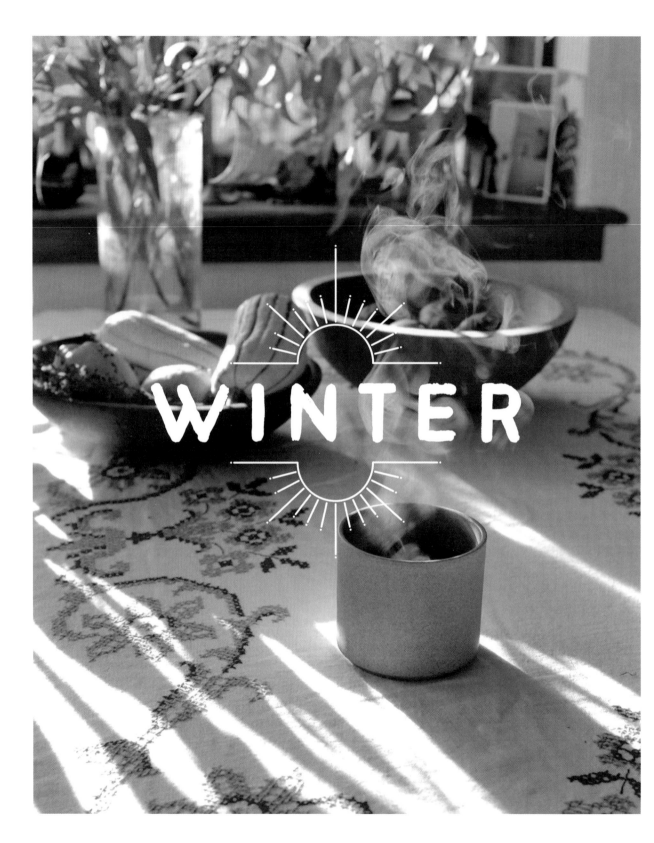

WINTER

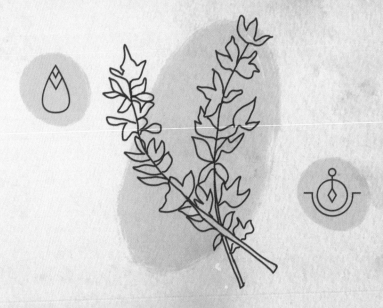

THE WINTER SEASON, WHEN WE'RE CELEBRATING MORE AND spending less time outdoors, is a time of mystery, magic, and inward reflection. It's important to rest, dream more, and bring some extra light into our practices. We like to bring some green inside by creating windowsill gardens or seasonal bouquets with branches and evergreen plants and by infusing celebratory meals with herbal medicine.

With the hustle of the holidays, it's easy to let practices fall to the wayside. We suggest focusing on rituals that feel simple and fun, such as infusing wines with adaptogenic herbs and creating decadent medicinal desserts. Use herbs that are warming and stimulating, as these actions help move the stagnant kapha energy that can sometimes feel overwhelming—as if you're stuck in the mud—during this season.

Think of warm, pungent herbs such as cayenne, ginger, rosemary, and thyme to promote circulation and immune health. Try adding in more roasted roots such as beets, carrots, turnips, and potatoes, which help keep us grounded and nourished. If you're feeling full or backed up from all the celebrations, make sure you're getting enough fiber and winter greens—think broccoli, cauliflower, and dark leafy greens.

This slow and dark season can be hard for all of us. Think of it as a time to reset and dream. Remember all you've accomplished and reward yourself with a spirit of gratitude. Envision a new year with goals that are evolved to who you are now. This is a wonderful time to use rooty adaptogens and nervines such as chamomile, lavender, lemon balm, and skullcap to help lighten the mood. Remember to support your heart and spirit and honor your body's need for a slower pace during this season.

FOODS	HERBS	RITUALS	REDUCE
Warming and stimulating cooked foods, such as broths, soups, and stews Lots of spices to support the circulatory system in staying warm Fermented veggies to stimulate the digestive system and support systems of elimination	Warming spices: black pepper, cardamom, cinnamon, ginger, horseradish, sumac Warming and mucus-clearing herbs: cayenne, garlic, rosemary, sage, thyme Warming and immune system–focused adaptogens: ashwagandha, astragalus, maca, reishi, shiitake	Warming Winter Salt Scrubs (page 244) Warm baths, saunas, steam rooms, and Herbal Steams (page 146) to stay warm and relaxed Dry Brushing (page 145) to support the lymphatic system Yoga to support the lymph and circulatory systems Breath work to stay embodied	Sweet, salty foods, and processed foods Wet, heavy, and dense foods, and foods that are high in saturated fats Cow dairy products Eating heavy meals and snacking throughout the day Eating and drinking as a way of coping emotionally Overextending yourself

WINTER SEASON

ELEMENTS: Water and earth

QUALITIES: Cold and wet

DOSHA: Kapha

BALANCING WINTER FLAVORS: Bitter, spicy, pungent, sour, sweet

SIGNALS OF BALANCE: Taking time to rest, filling your own cup first, having steady energy, eating to feel nourished but not full, maintaining a healthy immune system

SIGNALS OF IMBALANCE: Overcommitting, overindulging, depleted energy, stagnation, wet colds and flus, mucus in the respiratory system, heavy and sluggish digestion

Everyday Winter Berry Brew

Winter is a time to focus on warming and heart-centered herbs, so we can be merry, share love and gratitude, and bring all that goodness into the New Year. Hibiscus and rose hips support the heart, energetically and physically. Schisandra and elderberries support the immune system, and as an adaptogenic herb, schisandra promotes energy and stamina in the depths of winter. We also added a touch of ginger to the blend to keep circulation and energy moving.

FILLS 1 PINT-SIZED JAR

½ cup dried rose hips

½ cup dried hibiscus calyxes

¼ cup dried elderberries

¼ cup dried schisandra berries

2–3 tablespoons ground ginger

2 teaspoons dried licorice, optional

+ NOTE: All herbs should be cut and sifted.

Add herbs to a bowl or jar and mix well with a spoon. Store in a jar with a tight-fitting lid to keep the herbs fresh for use over the next couple weeks. Create a label for the jar, with details such as the date made and what herbs were used.

To make a daily quart of tea, add 2 to 3 tablespoons (about 1 teaspoon or more per cup) of the blend to a muslin bag or tea pouch and place inside a small pan, covered. Decoct the herbs (page 96) by slowly simmering them for at least 10 to 15 minutes. Take out the herbs and enjoy this tea throughout the day, adding honey or lemon to taste. We suggest sipping on about 2 to 4 cups throughout the day to get the most benefit. You can store in the fridge for up to 2 days. ∎

Minty Holiday Tea

This tea blend is the perfect holiday sweet treat when served hot and combined with honey. It's restorative and relaxing, with the help of nervous-system supportive lemon balm, which will curb holiday stress and tension. It's great to drink before a big gathering to calm down, or after a holiday meal to ease any bloating or indigestion that can occur after a holiday feast. The fennel and peppermint are both carminatives that help reduce bloating and cramping. But this blend is so refreshing and delicious that you and your guests will hardly care it's medicinal. FILLS 1 QUART-SIZED JAR

1 tablespoon dried rooibos

1 tablespoon dried lemon balm

½ teaspoon dried fennel seeds

2 teaspoons dried peppermint

+ NOTE: All herbs should be cut and sifted.

Blend together the dried herbs in a small bowl. Store in a labeled jar in a cool, dark place.

To use the tea, add 1 tablespoon or less per cup. Alternatively, enjoy this mix at a small gathering by adding all of the blend to a small teapot or quart-sized mason jar with 4 cups of boiling water. Make sure to warm the glass before adding in boiling water, to prevent breakage. Allow the tea to sit covered for 8 to 10 minutes, in order to infuse, and then strain and serve. Add honey to taste. ▪

Fire Cider Elixir

This immune-boosting fire cider tea is packed full of stimulating herbs to rev up the body's defenses, break up congestion, and fight colds. You can drink this mixture throughout the day when you're feeling under the weather. FILLS 2 QUART-SIZED JARS

2 quarts water

4-inch thumb fresh ginger, chopped

1 teaspoon roughly chopped fresh horseradish

2 garlic cloves, smashed

½ cup dried hibiscus calyxes

1 pinch ground cayenne

¼ cup raw local honey

Juice of 1 lemon

¼ cup apple cider vinegar

To a heavy-bottomed soup pot over low to medium heat, add the water, ginger, horseradish, garlic, hibiscus, and cayenne. Bring to a simmer and allow the mixture to decoct (page 96) for 20 to 30 minutes. Turn off the heat and strain out the herbs. Add in the honey, lemon juice, and apple cider vinegar. Taste and dilute with more water or add more sweetener, to your liking. If spicy peppers give you digestive system woes, simply remove the cayenne from the mix. ■

Ashwagandha Turmeric Golden Milk, page 187

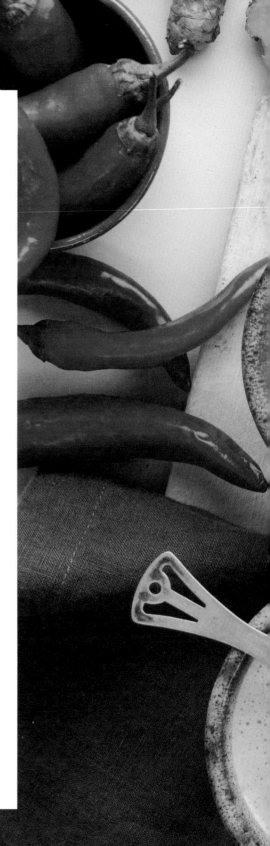

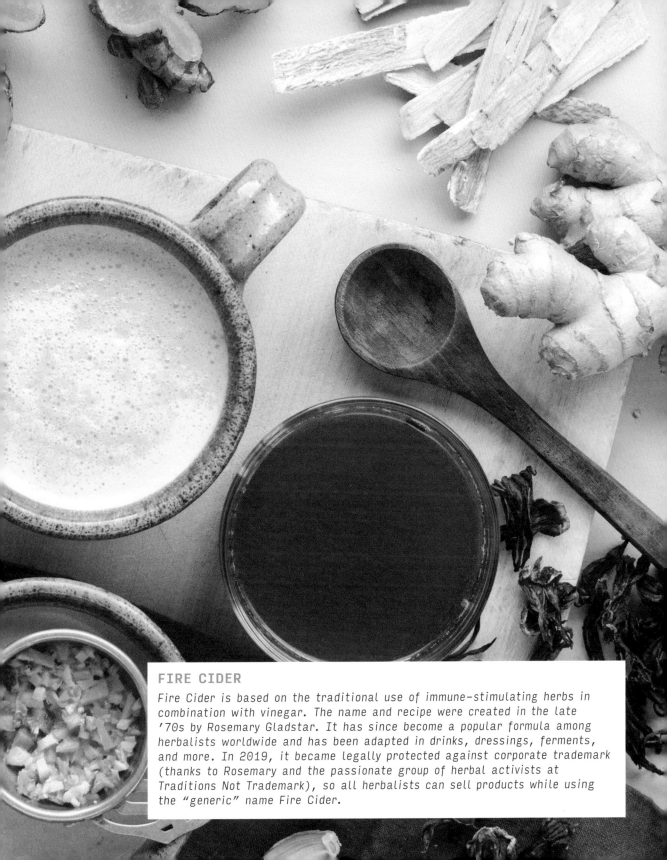

FIRE CIDER

Fire Cider is based on the traditional use of immune-stimulating herbs in combination with vinegar. The name and recipe were created in the late '70s by Rosemary Gladstar. It has since become a popular formula among herbalists worldwide and has been adapted in drinks, dressings, ferments, and more. In 2019, it became legally protected against corporate trademark (thanks to Rosemary and the passionate group of herbal activists at Traditions Not Trademark), so all herbalists can sell products while using the "generic" name Fire Cider.

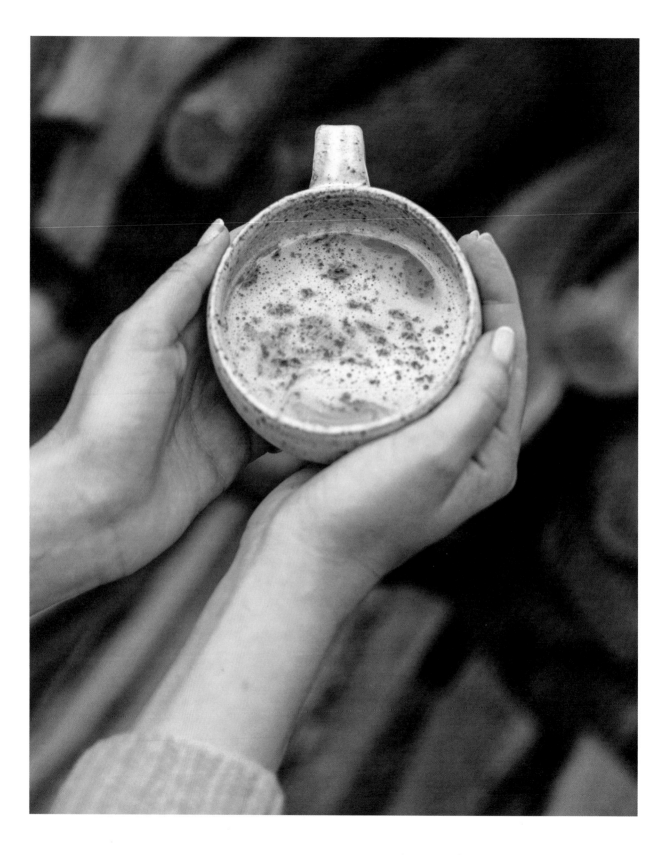

Spicy Mushroom Hot Cacao

Back when we first started The Kosmic Kitchen, we made small batches of a spicy mushroom cacao blend and sold them at a once-a-year holiday market in Orlando. Everyone loved it and still ask if we sell it to this day! This recipe will satisfy the spicy-mushroom-hot-cacao craving you didn't know you had. Sea salt is essential to smoothing out the bitterness of the chocolate and making sweet flavors more present, and a little pinch of flake salt on top when serving to add a decadent touch. Use whatever milk you prefer, though the slight bitterness of the pumpkin is nice here. Adjust the heat or sweet to your liking, and if you're up for it, hot cacao is always better with a dollop of freshly made whipped cream. SERVES 2

1 cup water

3 tablespoons cacao powder

2 teaspoons reishi powder, or a mushroom powder blend

1 cup pumpkin seed milk (see page 90) or homemade milk of choice

3 tablespoons maple syrup

3 ounces dark chocolate, roughly chopped

¼ teaspoon ground cinnamon

Pinch of ground cayenne

Pinch of flake salt, for garnish

Cacao powder, for garnish

In a saucepan, bring the water to a simmer on medium-high heat, then whisk in the cacao and reishi powders. Add in the pumpkin seed milk, maple syrup, dark chocolate, cinnamon, cayenne, and sea salt, whisking until the chocolate is melted and creamy, about 5 minutes. Divide between 2 mugs, sprinkle with flake salt, dust with cacao powder, and enjoy. ▪

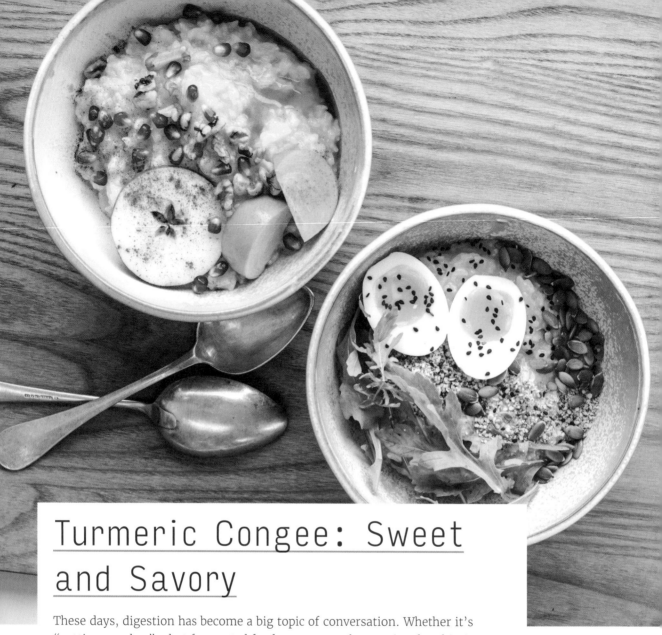

Turmeric Congee: Sweet and Savory

These days, digestion has become a big topic of conversation. Whether it's "getting regular," what fermented foods to eat, or what strain of probiotics are the best, people are talking about their guts and how to get them healthy. Something Chinese medicine and Asian cultures have been using for more than two thousand years is congee, or *jook*, a delicious, digestive-harmonizing dish of rice porridge.

Enjoying a warm bowl of congee for breakfast has become a Kosmic Kitchen staple. It can easily be prepared the night before or even overnight in a slow cooker. You can also water down leftover grains to create a batch of congee. Plus, congee is easy to digest, can be packed full of medicinal herbs, and is simply delicious. This porridge-like dish is warming and nourishing and perfect for those who are dry, depleted, or recovering from illness—or a hangover. We suggest the sweet option for those who need more of the moistening water element, and the savory for those who need more nourishment and fire element.

MAKES ABOUT 8 CUPS

1 cup basmati, brown, or jasmine rice

6 to 8 cups water

1 teaspoon ground turmeric

SWEET TOPPINGS

Toasted nuts or seeds, such as walnuts, pecans, or sunflower seeds

Seasonal berries and sliced fruits (can be stewed), such as persimmon, apple, or pear

Drizzle of maple syrup or sweetener of choice

SAVORY TOPPINGS

Toasted or black sesame seeds

Six-minute hard-boiled egg

Smoked salmon

Tamari or soy sauce

Dulse seaweed flakes

Seasonal sautéed or steamed greens, such as bok choy, spinach, or swiss chard

Roasted veggies, such as carrots or broccoli

Add the rice, water, and turmeric, if using, to a medium pot, bring to a boil on medium-high heat, then reduce heat to low (the lowest your stove can go) and let simmer for at least 2 hours. If time permits, consider cooking for 2 to 6 hours, since the longer the congee cooks, the more medicinal it becomes. You can also prepare the congee in your slow cooker by combining the ingredients and cooking at the low setting for 6 to 8 hours. ■

CONGEE

Traditionally, congee is eaten for breakfast and is part of a typical qing dan diet that consists of eating simple foods, "mostly grains, beans, vegetables, and fruits," according to Paul Pitchford, author of one of our favorite books, Healing with Whole Foods. He translates qing as "clear" or "pure and light," and dan as "bland." The foods that support this kind of diet are believed to be the foundation of good health and long life in Chinese medicine.

Chinese medicine practitioners and kitchen herbalists worldwide are known for adding herbs such as astragalus, jujube dates, and ashwagandha into congee and porridges as a way of "eating your medicine." A wide spectrum of common ailments can be supported with herbs and vegetables cooked in with the congee. A simple bowl of congee is a great way to give your digestion a break, which further promotes healing in the body. A good source for what specific plants to use is Healing with Whole Foods or The Book of Jook by Bob Flaws.

■ *For a warming and moistening porridge, great for vata constitutions, try: basmati rice, maca, ghee, honey, and stewed berries with spices.*

■ *For a cooling and cleansing porridge, great for pitta constitutions, try: quinoa, shatavari, steamed bitter greens, runny egg, and fresh herbs.*

■ *For a warming and cleansing porridge, great for kapha constitutions, try: millet, astragalus, fresh arugula, sliced radish, and smoked salmon.*

Ginger Pomegranate Molasses Hot Toddy

A folk remedy known to soothe sore throats, warm the body, and ward off sickness, there's nothing that hits the spot on a cold evening quite like a hot toddy. Pomegranate molasses has been used in Persian cuisine for thousands of years and is one of our favorite kitchen staples that adds a tangy sweet flavor to salad dressings, dips, and drinks. To add extra heat to this toddy, ginger and turmeric act as immune tonics and help bolster the body's ability to resist imbalances of the season. SERVES 2

2 cups water

½ teaspoon ground turmeric

1 teaspoon freshly grated ginger

1 tablespoon pomegranate molasses

2 teaspoons raw local honey

¼ cup brandy or rum

2 dropperfuls bitters of your choice, optional

2 lemon slices, for garnish

In a saucepan, warm the water over medium heat, whisking in the turmeric, ginger, and pomegranate molasses. Bring to a low simmer for about 5 minutes so flavors can meld. Remove the saucepan from the heat and stir in the honey and brandy. Divide between 2 mugs if desired, and add a dropperful of your favorite bitters in each mug. Serve with a slice of fresh lemon. ∎

Miso Immune Soup with Astragalus, Burdock, and Shiitake

The adaptogen astragalus has an affinity to the immune system. In Eastern medicine traditions, it's known as a chi, or energy, tonic. The root of astragalus strengthens digestion and supports the immune system, which makes it wonderful to use throughout the year or in times when your body feels run down and in need of extra support. SERVES 2 TO 3

4–6 cups water

1 burdock root, sliced

2 cups fresh shiitake mushrooms, chopped

1 bunch kale, shredded

One 14-ounce package firm tofu, cubed

4 Miso Immune Soup Balls (page 115)

1 carrot, thinly sliced

1 bunch green onions/scallions, white and tender pale green parts thinly sliced

In a saucepan, heat the water on medium high until it comes to a boil. Add the burdock root and shiitake mushrooms, reduce the heat to medium, and allow the mixture to simmer, covered, for at least 15 minutes, or until veggies are tender. As the burdock root and mushrooms cook, add in the kale and tofu, and allow to cook for the last 5 minutes. Just before you turn off the heat, add in the Miso Immune Soup Balls one by one to taste, using a whisk to quickly emulsify. Divide the soup between the bowls and top with the carrot and green onion slices. ■

Warm Delicata Squash and Kale Salad with Maca Miso Dressing

When delicata squash hits the farmers market, it's a welcome sight. Delicata is lovely to cook with not just for the rich creamy flavor but also for the minimal prep time, since the skins are edible and delicious. This warm salad is great when you want something filling but not too heavy during winter. It comes together quickly by having cooked rice and the Adaptogenic Ginger Maca Miso Dressing on hand. Play around with the flavor combinations and ingredients in this recipe. Swap chard or collards for kale or use another squash if you can't find delicata. SERVES 2 TO 4

1 delicata squash, seeds removed and cut into ¼-inch half moons

1 tablespoon Ghee (page 110), melted

Sea salt salt

2 cups rice, cooked

1 bunch kale, chopped, leaves and steams, divided

½ cup chopped parsley

1 tablespoon dried currants

¼ cup fresh pomegranate seeds

¼ cup toasted slivered almonds

¼ cup Adaptogenic Ginger Maca Miso Dressing (page 106)

Flake salt, for garnish

Olive oil, for garnish

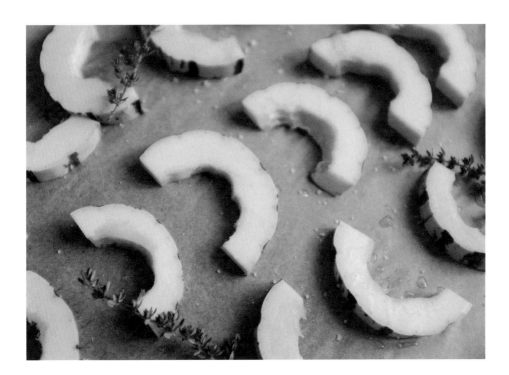

Preheat the oven to 350°F and line a baking sheet with parchment paper. Drizzle ghee over the squash and a sprinkle of sea salt, then toss with your hands or mix with a wooden spoon to coat evenly. Arrange the squash in an even layer on the baking sheet to roast for 15 to 20 minutes. Rotate the baking sheet halfway through roasting and flip the squash to ensure even cooking.

When the squash is almost done, heat a cast-iron skillet over medium heat, add the rice with a little ghee or water, and let it get crispy on the bottom, which should take about 4 minutes. Add the chopped kale stems to the rice to cook until they become tender, about 2 minutes. Toss in the kale leaves, cooking until wilted, about 1 minute. Once the squash is tender and beginning to brown, remove it from the oven to cool.

The trick to plating this salad is in the layering, so the kale greens continue to soften from the heat of the rice and squash. Use a platter or salad bowl and add half of each of the ingredients in this order: rice with kale stems and leaves, squash, parsley, currants, pomegranate seeds, toasted almonds, and the dressing. Repeat this process to form another layer and top it with a sprinkle of flake salt and a drizzle of olive oil. Enjoy this as a main dish or serve as a side dish. ▪

Comforting Chickpea Stew with Cardamom Basmati Rice

A warm pot of chickpeas simmering in spices is a delicious comfort food. This dish is easy to prepare and can be adapted depending on what you have in the fridge or pantry. When the chickpeas and rice are soaked overnight and you've got a jar of stock waiting in the fridge, this recipe comes together in no time at all. Stews and soups are a great way to get in immune-supporting roots such as astragalus or reishi mushroom. One thing to note with astragalus and most adaptogens is that they're best taken before getting sick with a cold or flu, since they tonify the body. SERVES 4 TO 6

FOR THE STEW

2 tablespoons coconut oil

2 teaspoons ground turmeric

1 teaspoon ground cinnamon

1 yellow onion, diced

2 garlic cloves, minced

3-inch thumb fresh ginger, minced

1 fennel bulb, chopped into ½-inch cubes

4 cups chickpeas, cooked

2 teaspoons sea salt

2 bay leaves

4 slices dried astragalus slices

One 14-ounce can diced tomatoes

3 cups Everyday Herbal Bone Broth (page 112), vegetable broth, or water

1 bunch greens, such as kale or collards, chopped into bite-sized pieces

½ bunch cilantro, roughly chopped, for garnish

FOR THE RICE

2 cups basmati rice, soaked (see page 88)

2 teaspoons ground cardamom

1 teaspoon sea salt

2 cups water

In a Dutch oven or heavy-bottomed soup pot, melt the coconut oil over medium heat. Sprinkle in the turmeric and cinnamon, stirring the spices into the coconut oil until fragrant, about 30 seconds. Toss in the onion and cook, covered, until tender and translucent, about 5 minutes. When the onions are soft, add in the garlic and ginger and cook until fragrant. Toss in the chopped fennel and chickpeas, sea salt, bay leaves, and astragalus slices and stir to incorporate, then cover with broth and add in the diced tomatoes. Bring to a simmer, then cover and reduce the heat to medium-low, cooking until the chickpeas are soft and the flavors meld, about 30 minutes.

As the stew is simmering, cook the rice. Add the soaked rice to a saucepan with a lid and sprinkle in the ground cardamom and salt, stirring to incorporate. Then pour in the water, cover, turn on the heat and bring to a boil, and then turn off the heat. Let the rice sit for about 15 minutes before removing the lid and fluffing the rice with a fork.

To finish the stew, stir in the greens during the last 5 minutes of cooking so they become tender. Remove bay leaves and astragalus slices. To serve, divide the cardamom rice between the bowls and top with a ladleful of stew. Garnish with plenty of cilantro leaves and enjoy hot. ■

Roasted Beet Hummus with Sumac and Seed Crackers

During the gray days of winter, this beet hummus adds a vibrant pop to any dish. The tangy, salty flavor of sumac—one of our favorite spices to sprinkle on everything from eggs to salads—adds a hit of salty and sour to your basic hummus recipe. Roasting a bunch of beets at the beginning of the week makes this recipe come together with little effort and relies on your food processor to do the work. The crackers are a riff on *Bon Appetit*'s addictive Seedy Oat Crackers. They're simple to make and full of wholesome seeds and oats, rather than flour. Enjoy them with dips or even crumbled and sprinkled on salads for a little crunch in the warmer months.

Roasted Beet Hummus

MAKES ABOUT 2 CUPS

1 beet, trimmed and washed (see note)

¼ cup plus 1 tablespoon olive oil

1½ cups chickpeas, cooked

2 garlic cloves, minced

1 tablespoon tahini

½ tablespoon pomegranate molasses, optional

½ teaspoon sumac, plus more for garnish

Juice of 1 lemon

¼ teaspoon sea salt

+ NOTE: This recipe only uses one roasted beet, but we recommend roasting a whole bunch of beets along with the one needed for this recipe. The roasting instructions below work for any type of vegetable.

Preheat the oven to 350°F and line a baking sheet with parchment paper. Place the beets on the prepared baking sheet and rub them with 1 tablespoon of olive oil. Roast until tender and easily pierced with a fork, 20 to 30 minutes. Remove from the oven when done and let cool. Save all but one beet for later.

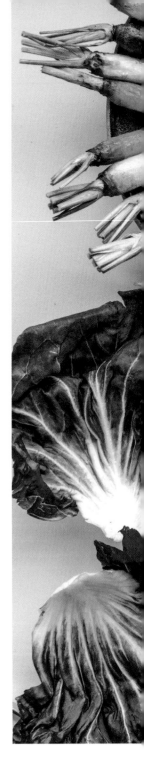

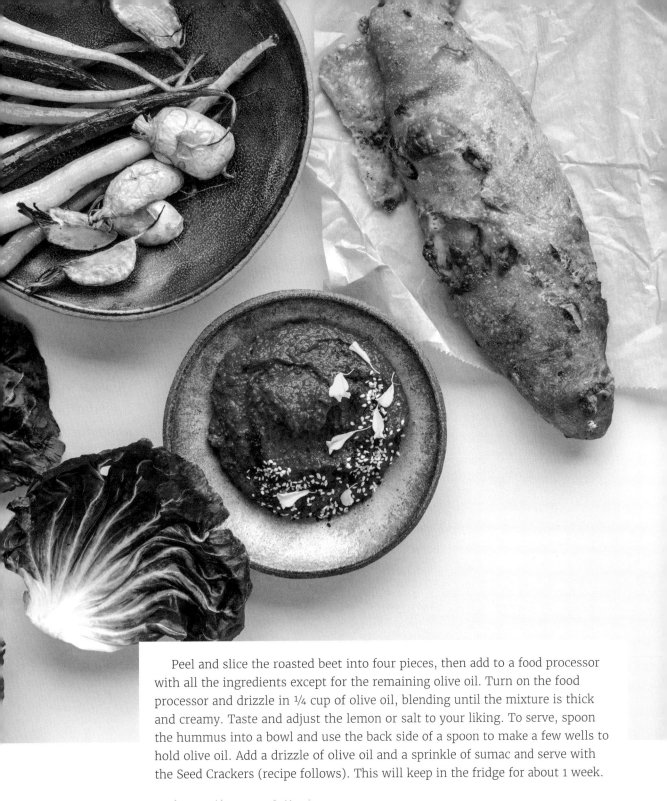

Peel and slice the roasted beet into four pieces, then add to a food processor with all the ingredients except for the remaining olive oil. Turn on the food processor and drizzle in ¼ cup of olive oil, blending until the mixture is thick and creamy. Taste and adjust the lemon or salt to your liking. To serve, spoon the hummus into a bowl and use the back side of a spoon to make a few wells to hold olive oil. Add a drizzle of olive oil and a sprinkle of sumac and serve with the Seed Crackers (recipe follows). This will keep in the fridge for about 1 week.

recipe continues on following page

Seed Crackers

SERVES 4

1 cup rolled oats

¾ cup raw pumpkin seeds

¼ cup raw sunflower seeds

¼ cup hemp seeds

¼ cup flax seeds

¼ cup sesame seeds

2 tablespoons poppy seeds

1 tablespoon minced fresh rosemary

1 teaspoon freshly cracked black pepper

1 teaspoon sea salt

1 tablespoon coconut oil or Ghee (page 110)

1 tablespoon maple syrup

½ cup warm water

Flake salt

Preheat oven to 375°F and line a baking sheet with parchment paper. Cut out an additional piece of parchment paper the size of the baking sheet and set aside. In a small mixing bowl, add all dry ingredients and combine well. In a small saucepan over medium-low heat, melt the coconut oil and maple syrup together. Then in a separate mixing bowl, add the warm water and whisk in the melted coconut oil and maple syrup. Add the wet mixture to the dry ingredients, combining well with a wooden spoon. Let the dough rest for 5 to 10 minutes so the oats soak up the moisture.

Add the dough to the prepared baking sheet and form a mound. Take the other piece of parchment paper and place it on top. Using a rolling pin, gently flatten until the dough is about ⅛-inch thick, then slowly peel back the top layer of parchment paper, reserving the parchment paper. Sprinkle the dough with flake salt and bake for 15 to 20 minutes, or until the edges are golden, rotating the tray halfway through.

Carefully slide the parchment paper and cracker off the baking tray and onto a cutting board and place the reserved piece of parchment on top. Flip the cracker over carefully and slide it back onto the baking sheet, then slowly remove the top sheet of parchment. Sprinkle with flake salt and bake for another 15 to 20 minutes or until the middle is firm. Remove the cracker from the oven and let it cool for about 10 minutes before breaking into pieces. Serve with the roasted beet hummus. Store extra crackers in a tightly sealed container for up to 1 week. ∎

Cast-Iron Fruit Crumble with Thyme and Rosemary

We're not big on baking, but we do love quick and easy crumbles to savor the fruit of the season. Making a crumble in a cast-iron skillet feels more rustic, and it can be served right on the table with a big spoon so everyone can help themselves. The addition of fresh thyme and rosemary adds an unexpected savory element that steers the crumble away from being overly sweet.

SERVES 4 TO 6

1 cup rolled oats

½ cup walnuts

¼ cup pecans

2 tablespoons maca powder

½ cup maple syrup, divided

½ teaspoon sea salt

½ stick butter, chilled and cut into cubes (see note)

2 pounds (about 5 cups) winter fruit, such as pears, apples, or persimmons, cut into ½-inch cubes

5 sprigs fresh thyme, leaves removed

2 sprigs fresh rosemary, leaves removed and roughly chopped

½ teaspoon ground cinnamon

½ teaspoon ground ginger

+ NOTE: You can use ¼ to ½ cup coconut oil to replace the butter. Just make sure the coconut oil is cold, otherwise it will melt too quickly, making a less crumbly topping.

Preheat oven to 350°F and grease the inside of a 9-inch cast-iron skillet. In a food processor, pulse the oats, walnuts, pecans, maca, ¼ cup maple syrup, sea salt, and butter until the mixture forms clumps. Check to see if the mixture stays together when you pinch it. In a mixing bowl, toss the fruit with the thyme, rosemary, cinnamon, ginger, and ¼ cup maple syrup. Add the fruit mixture to the cast-iron skillet in an even layer, and then top the fruit evenly with the crumble mixture. Bake for 30 minutes, or until the fruit has released its juices and the top is golden brown. Serve warm. ■

Ginger Persimmon Oat Bars

This warming winter snack is the perfect way to incorporate your favorite dried fruits and berries. We use persimmons, as they grow prolifically out here in California, but feel free to use what is available where you live. Think about fruits such as dried pears, dates, and prunes, or even medicinal berries such as goji and hawthorn. The fresh ginger gives the bars an extra bite, and for good measure, this spice promotes circulation during the wet and cold season. MAKES 16 RECTANGULAR BARS

3½ cups rolled oats

1½ cups brown sugar

1¼ cups butter, room temperature

2 eggs

1½ tablespoons freshly grated ginger

½ tablespoon vanilla extract

2 teaspoons ground cinnamon

½ teaspoon sea salt

1 cup dried and chopped persimmons, or other seasonal fruit or herbal berries

⅔ cup roughly chopped walnuts, pumpkin seeds, or seed/nut of your choice

½ tablespoon black sesame seeds, for garnish

Preheat the oven to 350°F. Use a food processor to grind the oats finely, into a flour. To a mixing bowl, add the brown sugar and butter and blend with a mixer for a few minutes until they combine to create a smooth and velvety texture. Add in the eggs one at a time and mix on high, then drop the speed to low and add the grated ginger, vanilla extract, cinnamon, salt, and oat flour. Once smooth, fold in the dried fruit and chopped nuts or seeds.

    Scrape the mixture evenly into a square medium-sized baking pan lined with parchment paper, sprinkle the top with the black sesame seeds, and cook for 45 to 60 minutes or until the top turns a golden hue. Let the bake cool, store in the fridge covered (to keep them from drying out), and then cut into snack-sized squares to enjoy throughout the week. The bars will stay delicious for about a week when stored in an airtight container in the fridge. ∎

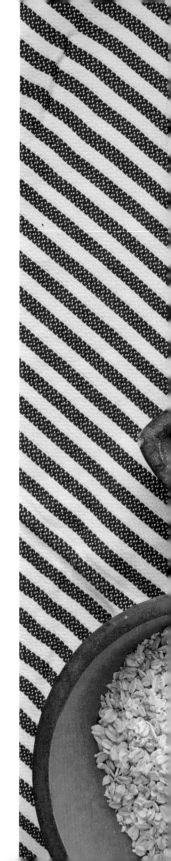

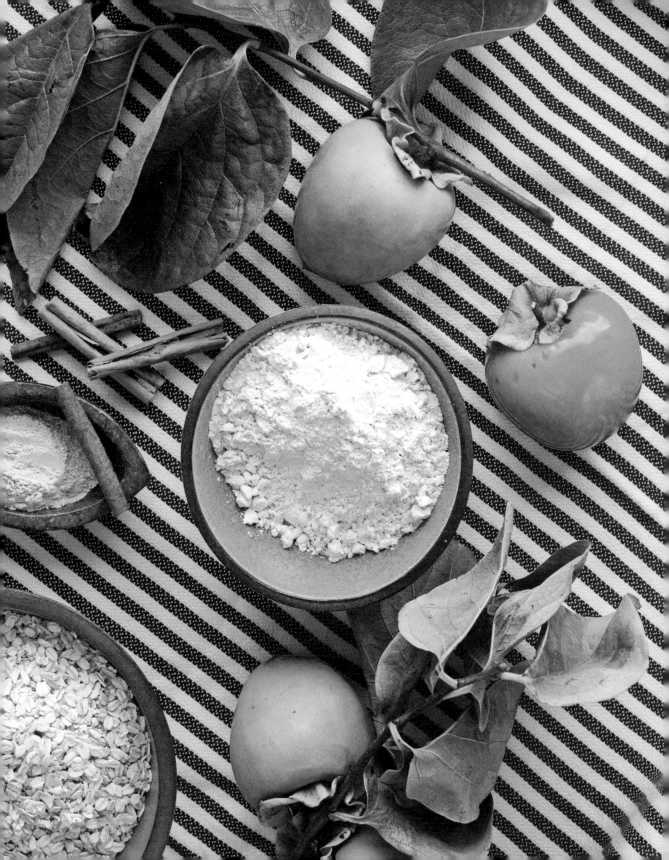

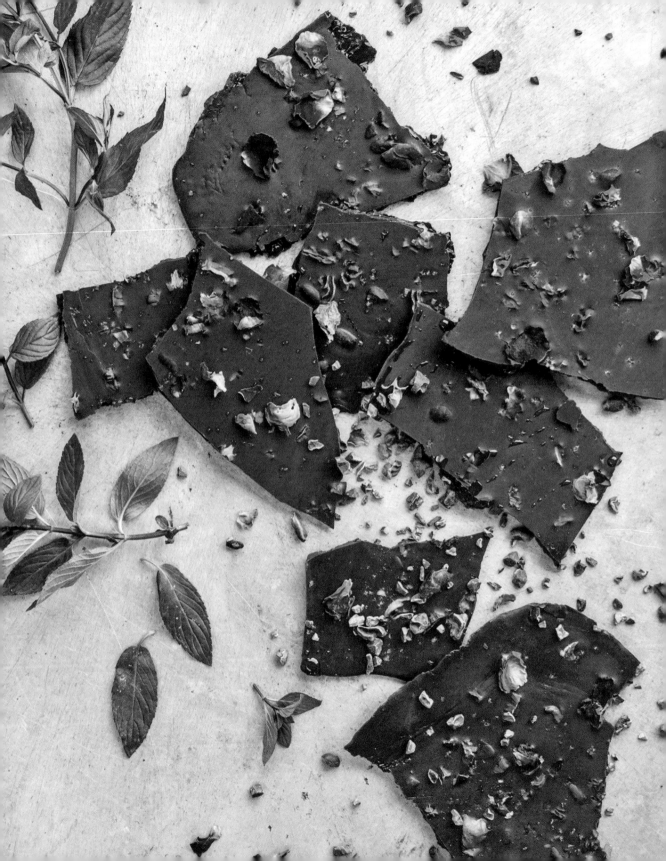

Reishi Rose Chocolate Bark

We can't seem to get enough of the magical combination that is reishi mushrooms and chocolate. This holiday bark is the perfect treat to satisfy those sweet cravings without needing to overindulge. Sea salt helps bring out the flavor of the chocolate, and the addition of the bitter cacao nibs keeps it from being overly sweet. Besides the reishi, we added a little ashwagandha to soothe our systems from the stress of the holiday season. While you might not want to share, this would be an easy last-minute homemade gift for any chocolate fan. SERVES 8

¼ cup coconut oil

¼ cup Ghee (page 110)

1 cup cacao powder

1 tablespoon reishi mushroom powder

2 teaspoons ashwagandha powder

1 teaspoon ground cardamom

2 tablespoons maple syrup

Sea salt

1 tablespoon cacao nibs

1 tablespoon dried rose petals

To a ceramic, glass, or other heatproof bowl, add the coconut oil and ghee and set over a simmering pot of water. You'll want the bowl to be large enough to sit on top of the pot and to hover above the water but not touch it. The goal is to make a double boiler. Stir until the fats have melted and are warm, then take the ceramic bowl off the pot of water. Set the bowl on a heatproof surface and whisk in the cacao, reishi, ashwagandha, cardamom, maple syrup, and a pinch of sea salt. Taste to make sure the sweetness and salt are to your liking and adjust as needed. Pour the mix into a 9 x 6 (or similar) glass or ceramic baking dish in an even layer, then sprinkle the cacao nibs and dried rose petals on top. You can also line a small baking sheet with parchment and pour the melted chocolate mixture into an even layer. Pop the bark into the freezer to set. The bark should be ready after 20 to 30 minutes. Remove it from the freezer and use a metal spatula or butter knife to break it up. To keep the bark firm, store in the freezer if not enjoying immediately. ■

Winter Rituals for Intentional Nourishment

As the days get darker and the cold weather sinks in, our bodies need time to rest. It's no surprise we naturally feel the urge to stay home and bundle up, surrounded by things that will keep us cozy. Simple things, such as going out and being social or even waking up at our normal time each morning, become harder to do. These are little messages from the body, asking us to take time to pause. Our bodies thrive with rest, relaxation, and alone time, though we barely allow ourselves those luxuries for fear of not doing enough or not being productive. It's usually when we haven't taken time for ourselves that we experience seasonal illness and we're forced to clear our schedules. While it's important to encourage warmth in the body and deep nourishment, sitting in the quiet space winter provides has profound effects on our spiritual and mental health.

While you'll likely be spending most nights during the winter at home, make sure to create intentional time for yourself. These rituals are meant to be a touchstone of creating space to honor the body, mind, and spirit. You can make them as simple or elaborate as you like, just remember the elemental aspects that will help bring you back into balance if you're feeling cold, congested, or sluggish. One of our favorite ways to enjoy an evening alone is by making a nourishing dinner, dimming the lights and burning beeswax candles, listening to soothing music, taking a bath, and getting to bed early so there's plenty of time to enjoy sleeping. Find ways to make these intentional nights by yourself a weekly ritual and you'll be surprised at how relaxed, rested, and connected you feel.

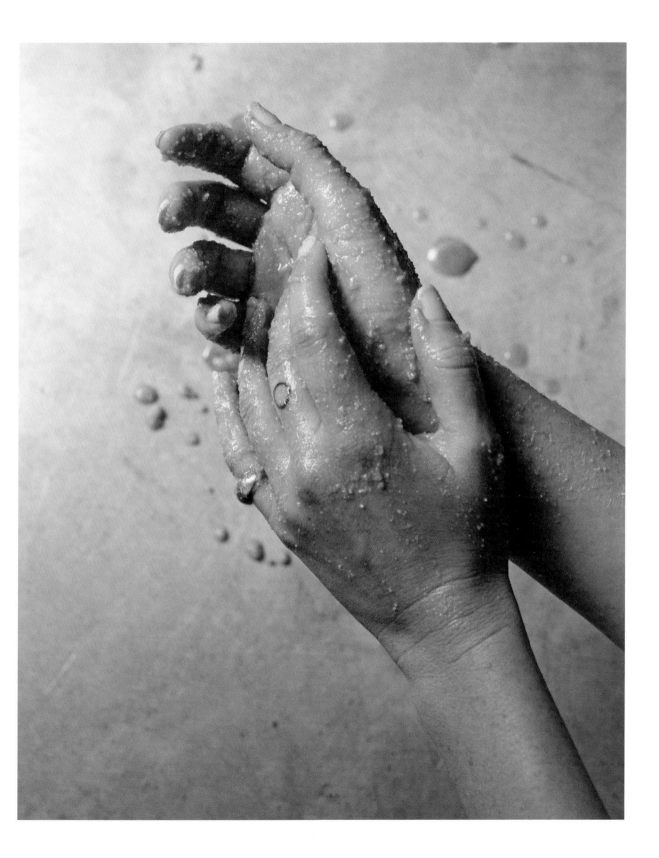

Warming Winter Salt Scrub

Treating ourselves to a weekly salt scrub has become one of our favorite rituals that feels luxurious while being inexpensive and simple to do. A salt scrub is both hydrating and exfoliating, and it promotes circulation and overall lymphatic health. Our teacher DeAnna Batdorff turned us on to the benefits of supporting our lymphatic system and how deeply it's woven into the fabric of our immune system—in fact, it actually is our immune system! In the heart of winter or any time of stagnation, it's important to make scrubbing and circulation-pumping activities nonnegotiable rituals. This is especially important for those who run cold and wet, such as vata and kapha doshas. MAKES 1 SALT SCRUB

¼ to ½ cup finely ground sea salt

½ to 1 cup sunflower, sesame, or other oil

Sunflower oil is tridoshic, meaning good for all body types, but we prefer to use sesame in winter, as it's warming by nature. You can also use an infused herbal oil to soak in added benefits. Mix the salt and oil in a jar or small bowl to form a thick paste to the texture of your liking, making sure it's not so oily that the salt doesn't exfoliate and not so salty that it's too exfoliating or rough.

To use the scrub, stand on a towel in your bathroom and apply the oil starting at your feet and working in upward motions toward your heart. Scrub until the skin turns pink, which indicates that fresh blood is coming to the surface of the skin. Work your way up vigorously as this helps to pump the lymph and get your circulation moving. Gently scrub your neck and face, if you feel called to, though that can be irritating for some. Finally, get into your bath carefully (be careful not to slip), and try to focus on your breath for 10 to 15 minutes. ∎

Warming Herbal Foot Soak

While a footbath may seem too simple to be effective, it's incredibly transformative over time, especially when done 2 to 3 times a week. Many Chinese medicine practitioners recommend herbal footbaths to be done almost every day during the fall and winter seasons, as it helps protect the body and build up defenses during the colder seasons. This herbal practice has been traditionally prepared with plants from around the world, as it's an easy way to get herbs quickly into the body and to relax the nervous system.

Basil	Lavender	Rosemary
Chamomile	Lemon balm	Skullcap
Cinnamon	Mugwort	Thyme
Ginger	Peppermint	

Try one or a combination of the herbs above. Use warming herbs in your blend—such as cinnamon, ginger, rosemary, and mugwort—to promote circulation during the depths of winter. Use about ½ to 1 cup of dried, cut, and sifted herbs per foot soak. Put the herbs into a large basin, pour over boiling water, and wait about 15 minutes or so for the mixture to become comfortable enough to place your feet in.

Soak your feet while meditating, reading a book, or engaging in another relaxing activity. Allow this to be a time for yourself to rejuvenate and to call in abundant and healing energy. ∎

NOTES OF GRATITUDE

Note from Sarah

I feel so honored to have been able to go through the creation of this cookbook with my longtime friend and business partner, Summer. We have seen each other through many transitions, and it makes me so proud to know we created something we truly love with each other. Summer, you constantly inspire me, and I can't think of a better person to bring my dreams to life with.

To my mother, who has been my angel, my best friend, and the image of the person I want to become: your unyielding love and support have given me the confidence I didn't know I had to do things only you knew I could do. I feel so lucky to call you my mama. To Ray, for giving us the most beautiful life filled with fun, adventure, and animals. I feel so grateful to call you my dad and to have your support in my life.

To August, my partner and lover, thank you for being by my side throughout the journey that is writing a cookbook, even though it hasn't always been easy. It brings me so much joy to be growing together in our work and passions to help the world be a better place. You inspire me endlessly with what you've been able to create and how much you've grown into yourself.

To Lisa and RoseAnn, I feel so much gratitude for your presence in my life and the beauty you both share with all of us. I have deeply appreciated your support and love over the past few years as you've welcomed me into your family.

To my Orlando community, far and wide, how can I even begin to put into words the magic we all created together? I am forever in awe of that time, how much love the plants brought out in us to share wherever we go, and who I was able to become because of that. You're my family and soul mates. To my OAEC community, what an incredible place we all get to be in together, nourishing change makers in the world. You've forever inspired me with what can be accomplished by a group of heart-centered people who created a living sanctuary honoring Mother Nature.

To my teachers, Tina Richards, Emily Ruff, Mark Disharoon, Rosemary Gladstar, Candis Cantin, Kathleen Harrison, DeAnna Batdorff: What a gift to have been in your presence and to be able to carry on the teachings that have changed so many lives. Thank you for sharing your light with us all. A special thanks to DeAnna Batdorff and Zoë Gardner for taking the time to put your skilled and thoughtful eyes on our manuscript. It means so much to us.

To Juree, our editor, for being our biggest cheerleader along the way and being such a joy to work with. To our team at Roost, thank you for believing in us, holding our vision, and helping us create our first cookbook. To Amy, for this super special and unique interior design—we love it. To our students and Kosmic Kitchen community of plant lovers, thank you for your continuous support and courage to be on a path of healing and self-discovery. You're why we do what we do. ▪

Note from Summer

To the plants, thank you for guiding me to this work, and for healing me.

To Sarah, thank for your teaching me to live in my power. For supporting me and cocreating with me. I'm so honored to work alongside you, to call you my best friend (though you are so much more than that), and I'm forever inspired by your magnetic creativity and authenticity.

To all my teachers, thank you for sharing your craft so generously and for your commitment to healing. Tina, every garden I grow is infused with your healing essence. Emily, thank you for showing me that herbalism isn't just about healing ourselves, it's about being an activist for the land and its people. Rosemary, thank you for cultivating the seed of herbalism within me, and for teaching so many of us how to live in relationship with the Earth. DeAnna, thank you for your depth of commitment to Ayurveda and the art of healing. Your teachings have inspired so much of our work and this cookbook. Zoë, thank you for your tireless research into plant safety and formulation, your friendship, and for your time and energy on this book.

To my family, you've always supported my adventures and studies, no matter how wild. Thank you all for being so open-minded and intellectually curious. Dad, thank you for teaching me about the trees and showing me how to find freedom in the outdoors. Mom, thank you for always reminding me that it's more fun to be different.

To Jacqueline, my soul sister. Thank you for finding me in this life, over and over again. You make life more joyous. I couldn't have finished these recipes without our kitchen dance sessions powering me through.

To our Orlando community, there are no words to explain the magic we shared. The roots we planted together are the foundation of this cookbook and my life as a whole. Thank you for teaching me how to live a more embodied life.

To Jorge, my love. Thank you for being a wellspring of support. For lifting me up and seeing me. You're an incredible human and creator. Thank you for capturing us in our element through your photography.

To Alysia, Anna-Alexia, Juree, and the whole Roost team, thank you for believing in us and helping to bring our vision to life. And a special shout out to Amy, who went above and beyond with the amazing design of this book.

To our students and community, thank you for supporting our work. We are endlessly grateful. Because of you we are able to bring our passions to life. ▪

KOSMIC KITCHEN RESOURCES

"Herbal education begins with changing our consciousness."

—PAM MONTGOMERY

Where to Buy Herbs

Something we always get asked is, "Where do I buy herbs?" While there are a few staple companies such as Mountain Rose Herbs for bulk and Traditional Medicinals for tea, there are also a lot of different standards. Between FairWild, fair trade, and pharmacopoeial, you might be wondering, "What does it all mean?!"

In this book we wanted to focus on products that can be bought easily across the country, on the regular. Things that are affordable and accessible. However, there are many amazing boutique herbal companies, and we encourage you to buy local whenever possible. It's also ideal to connect with a local community or clinical herbalist, as they can come up with a formula unique to your energetics and ecosystem.

We also recognize that these standards can make buying herbs costly, so some smaller companies and local farms opt out. It's best to ask folks what their practices are; this dialogue promotes mindful practices, whether they are currently implementing them or not. Consumer-driven change can happen, so be sure to reach out, ask questions, tell companies what you would like to see, and support businesses that care.

BULK AND DRIED HERBS

If you're looking for dried herbs, so you can make your own teas and use adaptogens on the regular, we highly suggest sourcing from Mountain Rose Herbs. They buy organic herbs, hire herbalists, support herbal education, and have a strong commitment to sustainability.

ESSENTIAL OILS

Buying cheap essential oils is tempting, but this matters almost more than where you buy your dried herbs. For instance, it can take from 30 to 100-plus plants to make just 1 drop of essential oil. Think about how many resources were used to create that medicine, and how important it is that these plants were cultivated mindfully. Essential oils are a hyperpotent form of plant medicine that should be used and made wisely. We suggest Simplers Botanicals, Veriditas, Pranarōm, Mountain Rose Herbs, or Aura Cacia.

Using hydrosols, the by-product of making essential oils through distillation, is a wonderful way to enjoy the benefits of potent plant properties while using far less plant matter to create them. These aromatic plant waters are a luxurious and gentle treatment for healing the skin and can be used as a refreshing mist year-round but especially in the warmer months.

GROW YOUR OWN

Nothing compares to growing your own herbs. We suggest seeds from Strictly Medicinals or getting them sourced locally from a seed exchange or starts from a local plant nursery. We're lucky enough to live near the Sonoma County Herb Exchange, so we get a ton of our medicine grown fresh from local farmers.

HERBAL PILLS

Gaia does such a wonderful job at making compounded formulas that are easy to use and effective. They also have a farm, in North Carolina, and hire herbalists. On their farm they weave in agroforestry and beekeeping, and they're passionate about regenerative practices in general. We recommend trying their herb pills if you're less inclined to make tea or take a tincture every day.

HERBAL POWDERS

We suggest buying from Mountain Rose Herbs, Frontier Co-op, or better yet, at your local herb shop. We love buying a 1-pound bag of herbs we use frequently, so we always have some handy.

HERBAL TEAS

For on the go, Traditional Medicinals teas are the best. They have a team of plant lovers and herbalists across all departments, from sourcing and formulating to marketing. We love that a full box of tea is just around five bucks, organic whenever possible, and available in both local co-ops and big-box stores such as Whole Foods and Target. Their teas are almost all pharmacopoeial grade, meaning their herbs are pharmacy grade, tested, and are sure to work. Plus, their foundation's mission is to support communities where their herbs are cultivated or collected.

HERBAL TINCTURES

Herb Pharm is one of the few US herbal companies that actually has their own farm and an educational program for budding herbalists at their headquarters in Oregon. Tinctures are great for when you're on the go, and they work almost instantaneously. Herb Pharm is also committed to sustainability, mindful sourcing, and effective formulas.

MUSHROOMS

We swear by anything made by Paul Stamets at Host Defense. His capsules and tinctures are made from mushroom cultivars that are grown in-house, and they utilize mycelium to create mushroom medicines that are incredibly potent and bioavailable. You can also buy mushroom powders at Mountain Rose Herbs.

SEAWEEDS

We buy local through Strong Arm Farm in California, but we also buy from Maine Coast Sea Vegetables, who sources sustainably off the Atlantic coastline.

Standards and Labels to Look For

BIODYNAMIC

A label that ensures the plants were grown in accordance with nature's natural cycles, with some unique (but cool) rituals involved. It's rooted in the teachings of Dr. Rudolf Steiner, who is also the father of Waldorf education. It addresses everything from healthy compost and soil rotation to proper and mindful integration of farm animals. Biodiversity is key in this practice.

DOSAGE INFORMATION

If you're using an herb for a desired medicinal effect, it's important to get the right dose. Many people think herbs don't work because they get a poor-quality product, or they try it once and it doesn't work due to lack of consistency. Be sure to investigate the required dosage by checking the supplement facts panel, a trusted herb book, or by looking up the plant "monographs" online.

FAIR TRADE

This global standard supports farmers and supplier communities worldwide. This certification ensures that people are getting fair wages, sometimes housing, and funds to support their local communities. It focuses on empowering both the workers and healthy environments.

FAIRWILD

This certification makes sure that herbs and other plants are wild-collected in a sustainable way that supports the local bioregion and collectors. Many herbs, such as wild American ginseng, are harvested and collected in such a way that puts the species in a very vulnerable position. We can't wait to see this label on more products!

FOREST GROWN

Plants are best grown in ecosystems, and this is truly what regenerative farming is all about. Monocropping plants, even if it's organic, doesn't build ecosystems or create rich habitats for other species to thrive. This new Forest Grown label is something to look out for in the future.

NON-GMO

This indicates that the plants are not made from genetically modified organisms, which create a whole world of issues for ecosystems and farmers. GMOs are a threat to our planet's biodiversity, and the term identifies plants as corporations' intellectual property. Most herbs don't have a GMO counterpart, but it's nice to know that companies are taking a stance with this label.

ORGANIC

Organic-certified plants are grown with no synthetic pesticides or fertilizers, no GMOs, and with soil health in mind. This is the easiest and best label to look for, if you're just looking for one.

PHARMACOPOEIAL GRADE

When something meets the standards of the United States Pharmacopoeia (USP), you will sometimes see it on the front of the label, but always on the supplement facts panel with a USP mark. This basically means that the herbs work. These plants have been rigorously tested to ensure they have enough active constituents that have been identified as medicinal markers by the USP. For example, chamomile products would need to be made from just the flowering tops and have enough volatile essential oils to be considered medicinal.

UNITED PLANT SAVERS

Members of United Plant Savers acknowledge and adhere to up-to-date standards on which plants should be avoided or carefully procured in commerce. United Plant Savers works diligently to determine which plants are at risk in North America of becoming extinct, especially due to overuse in commerce by the supplement/cosmetic industry. Some examples of plants that are particularly popular and need to be mindfully purchased (and used) or even swapped out for other alternatives are American ginseng, osha root, and white sage.

Further Education

AMERICAN HERBALIST GUILD

This association is the premiere guild for herbalists practicing and teaching in the United States. Here you can find practitioners and schools in your area.

www.americanherbalistsguild.com

CALIFORNIA SCHOOL OF HERBAL STUDIES

One of the oldest Western herbalism schools still standing, California School of Herbal Studies (CSHS) is recognized as one of the most prestigious and authentic herbal schools in the country. Founded by Rosemary Gladstar, this program has an incredible list of resident and guest teachers. The school also has an incredible garden with a few hundred species of medicinal plants and a robust lab to practice medicine making. They offer an immersive Roots and Intermediate program, medicine making courses, and more that take place in the countryside of Sonoma County. It's one of our favorite local herb schools to attend and teach at.

www.cshs.com

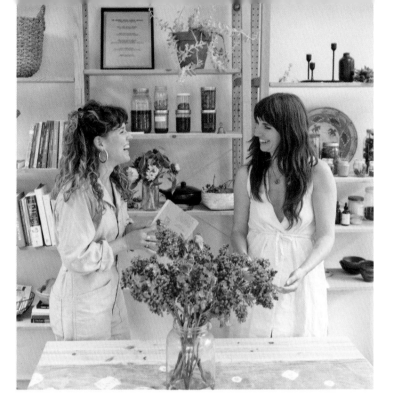

THE DHYANA CENTER

The dhyana Center, which is run by our amazing teacher DeAnna Batdorff, is one of our favorite schools. It has a full clinical Ayurvedic program, along with peripheral courses on everything from pulse taking to Ayurvedic cooking. You can also gain NAMA Ayurvedic accreditation over time by working as a student in their on-site clinic in Sebastopol, California.

www.dhyanacenter.com

FLORIDA SCHOOL OF HOLISTIC LIVING

With a hub in Orlando and satellite schools across the state, Florida School of Holistic Living (FSHL) offers dynamic herbalism classes that infuse Western herbal plants with tropical plant allies that grow in this unique subtropical ecosystem. Our mentor and teacher Emily Ruff runs the school that offers beginner programs all the way to community herbalist trainings. She also leads the Florida Herbal Conference that takes place each year in February.

www.holisticlivingschool.org

HERB PHARM HERBACULTURE INTERNSHIP PROGRAM

Want to learn more about growing plants and making medicine? This competitive internship program is offered during the summer months in Oregon. There you can work on one of Herb Pharm's main farms and learn about plant medicine from their local herbalists and farmers.

www.herb-pharm.com/connect/internship

THE KOSMIC KITCHEN ONLINE LEARNING

We offer online courses on elemental herbalism that highlight kitchen medicine practices. You can learn how to more deeply identify with energetics, develop kitchen skills, and make and infuse herbal medicines into everyday life. You can sign up for our e-mail list to be notified of upcoming programs.

www.thekosmickitchen.com

NATIONAL AYURVEDIC MEDICAL ASSOCIATION

National Ayurvedic Medical Association (NAMA) is North America's Ayurvedic certification and accreditation board. On their site you can look up programs across the continent (and online) that offer Ayurvedic studies.

www.ayurvedanama.org

THE SCIENCE AND ART OF HERBALISM CORRESPONDENCE COURSE

Our teacher Rosemary Gladstar has run this comprehensive herbal correspondence course for decades now. It covers all the body systems, herbs, and medicine making. There's homework and direct feedback from her team.

scienceandartofherbalism.com

UNITED PLANT SAVERS INTERNSHIPS AND PROGRAMS

United Plant Savers ensures that we can continue to use plant medicine for generations to come by protecting and cultivating at-risk herbal species in North America. They offer internships and programs to learn more about herbs and conservation, usually located in their Ohio plant sanctuary.

www.unitedplantsavers.org

Books We Love

COOKBOOKS

Fallon, Sally, and Mary G. Enig. *Nourishing Traditions: The Cookbook That Challenges Politically Correct Nutrition and the Diet Dictocrats.* Washington, DC: NewTrends Publishing, 2001.

Flaws, Bob. *The Book of Jook: Chinese Medicinal Porridges—A Healthy Alternative to the Typical Western Breakfast.* Boulder, CO: Blue Poppy Press, 2001.

Katz, Sandor Ellix. *The Art of Fermentation: An In-Depth Exploration of Essential Concepts and Processes from Around the World.* White River Junction, VT: Chelsea Green, 2012.

Madison, Deborah. *Vegetable Literacy: Cooking and Gardening with Twelve Families from the Edible Plant Kingdom, with Over 300 Deliciously Simple Recipes.* Berkeley, CA: Ten Speed Press, 2013.

McBride, Kami. *The Herbal Kitchen: Bring Lasting Health to You and Your Family with 50 Easy-to-Find Common Herbs and Over 250 Recipes.* Newburyport, MA: Conari Press, 2019.

Pitchford, Paul. *Healing with Whole Foods: Asian Traditions and Modern Nutrition.* Berkeley, CA: North Atlantic Books, 1996.

Swanson, Heidi. *Super Natural Every Day: Well-Loved Recipes from My Natural Foods Kitchen.* Berkeley, CA: Ten Speed Press, 2011.

GENERAL AYURVEDA

Frawley, David, and Vasant Lad. *The Yoga of Herbs: An Ayurvedic Guide to Herbal Medicine.* Twin Lakes, WI: Lotus Press, 1986.

Lad, Vasant. *Ayurveda: The Science of Self-Healing—A Practical Guide.* Twin Lakes, WI: Lotus Press, 2004.

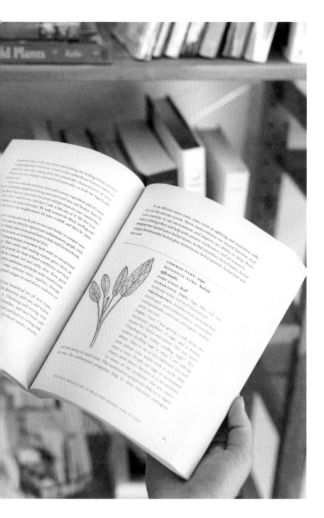

Hoffmann, David. *Medical Herbalism: The Science and Practice of Herbal Medicine*. Rochester, VT: Healing Arts Press, 2003.

Phillips, Nancy, and Michael Phillips. *The Herbalist's Way: The Art and Practice of Healing with Plant Medicines*. White River Junction, VT: Chelsea Green, 2005.

Tierra, Michael, and David Frawley. *Planetary Herbology: An Integration of Western Herbs into the Traditional Chinese and Ayurvedic Systems*. Twin Lakes, WI: Lotus Press, 1992.

Wood, Matthew. *The Practice of Traditional Western Herbalism: Basic Doctrine, Energetics, and Classification*. Berkeley, CA: North Atlantic Books, 2004.

MEDICINE MAKING

Cech, Richo, and Sena Cech. *Making Plant Medicine*. Williams, OR: Herbal Reads, 2016.

Green, James. *The Herbal Medicine–Maker's Handbook: A Home Manual*. Berkeley, CA: Crossing Press, 2000.

PLANT SPIRIT MEDICINE

Cowan, Eliot. *Plant Spirit Medicine: The Healing Power of Plants*. Columbus, NC: Granite Publishing, 1996.

Harrod Buhner, Stephen. *The Lost Language of Plants: The Ecological Importance of Plant Medicines to Life on Earth*. White River Junction, VT: Chelsea Green, 2002.

Wall Kimmerer, Robin. *Braiding Sweetgrass: Indigenous Wisdom, Scientific Knowledge, and the Teachings of Plants*. Minneapolis: Milkweed Editions, 2015.

Tiwari, Maya. *Ayurveda: A Life of Balance*. Rochester, VT: Healing Arts Press, 1995.

Tiwari, Maya. *The Path of Practice: The Ayurvedic Book of Healing with Food, Breath, and Sound.* Delhi: Motilal Banarsidass, 2002.

GENERAL HERBALISM

Gladstar, Rosemary. *Herbal Healing for Women*. New York: Fireside, 1993.

Gladstar, Rosemary. *Rosemary Gladstar's Herbal Recipes for Vibrant Health: 175 Teas, Tonics, Oils, Salves, Tinctures, and Other Natural Remedies for the Entire Family*. North Adams, MA: Storey Publishing, 2008.

Index

Entries in **bold** refer to overviews.

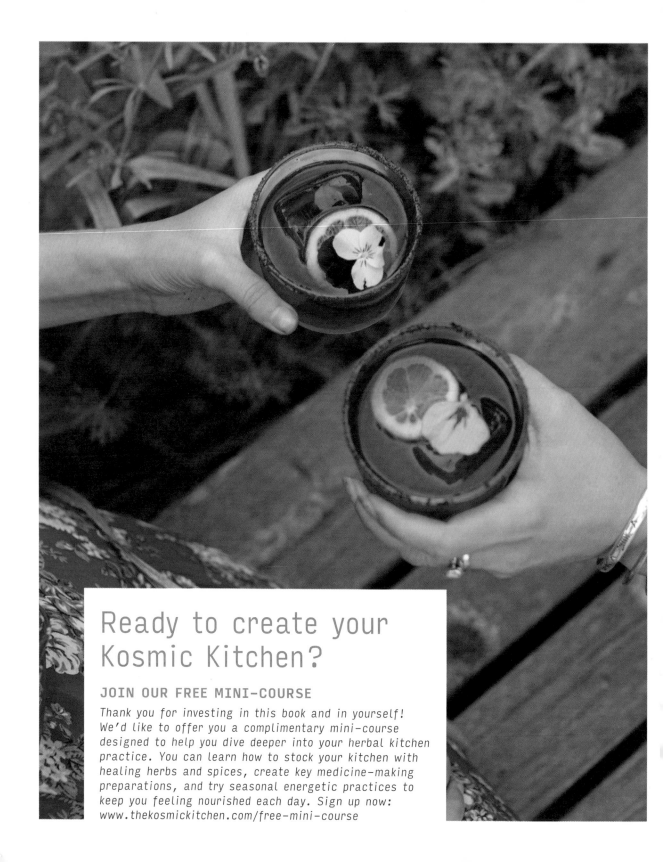

Ready to create your Kosmic Kitchen?

JOIN OUR FREE MINI-COURSE

Thank you for investing in this book and in yourself! We'd like to offer you a complimentary mini-course designed to help you dive deeper into your herbal kitchen practice. You can learn how to stock your kitchen with healing herbs and spices, create key medicine-making preparations, and try seasonal energetic practices to keep you feeling nourished each day. Sign up now: www.thekosmickitchen.com/free-mini-course